your
blueprint
for
pleasure

your
blueprint
for
pleasure

Discover THE 5 EROTIC TYPES
to Awaken—and Fulfill—Your Desires

JAIYA

UNION SQUARE & CO.

NEW YORK

UNION
SQUARE
&CO.

NEW YORK

ISBN 978-1-4549-5003-5
ISBN 978-1-4549-5004-2 (e-book)

Library of Congress Cataloging-in-Publication Data

Names: Jaiya, author.
Title: Your blueprint for pleasure : discover the 5 erotic types to awaken-and
fulfill-your desires / Jaiya.
Description: New York : Union Square & Co., [2023] | Includes bibliographical references and
index. | Summary: "Sexologist Jaiya has identified five erotic types that empower people with
the understanding that we are each erotically gifted and that our differences are our
strengths. Jaiya's framework will help readers bridge the sexual incompatibility gap,
become masters of their own sexual desire, and experience the deeper connection
and sexual satisfaction that they crave"— Provided by publisher.
Identifiers: LCCN 2023023009 (print) | LCCN 2023023010 (ebook) |
ISBN 9781454950035 (paperback) | ISBN 9781454950042 (ebook)
Subjects: LCSH: Sex. | Sexual health. | Sex (Psychology) | Interpersonal relations. |
BISAC: BODY, MIND & SPIRIT / Sacred Sexuality | HEALTH & FITNESS / Sexuality
Classification: LCC HQ21 .J29 2023 (print) | LCC HQ21 (ebook) | DDC 306.7—dc23/eng/20230713
LC record available at https://lccn.loc.gov/2023023009
LC ebook record available at https://lccn.loc.gov/2023023010

For information about custom editions, special sales, and premium purchases,
please contact specialsales@unionsquareandco.com.

Printed in Canada

2 4 6 8 10 9 7 5 3 1

unionsquareandco.com

Cover design by Elizabeth Mihaltse Lindy
Cover art © 2023 Petites Luxures
Interior design by Christine Heun
Icons by SeamlessPatterns/Shutterstock.com

This book is dedicated to the untamed wild ones, to those who know that authentic pleasure and ecstasy are the path to ultimate freedom, awakening, and love.
Thank you for being you.

And deep dedication and devotion to my dearest beloveds, Ian, Christian, Jon, and Michael Ashley—thank you for your undying support and unconditional love.

contents

FOREWORD
BY REGENA THOMASHAUER

It's a nearly impossible endeavor to *human* well. To connect deeply. To sex generously. To live with passion, fullness, humanity, humility, wisdom, and boundless gratitude.

We are all searching for liberation, to grow beyond our limitations, to become better versions of ourselves. Personally, I know I need all the help I can get.

True growth and expansion are immensely difficult precisely because they require befriending the parts of ourselves that have been rejected, forgotten, or banished by a patriarchal world culture that is invested in keeping us small and controlled.

As psychologist Karen Horney said, "You need not, and in fact cannot, teach an acorn to grow into an oak tree, but when given a chance, its intrinsic potentialities will develop."

All the acorn needs is a chance. Jaiya is that chance for us human beings.

Her journey of liberation and expansion creates a portal for each of us to find our *own* way.

Jaiya brilliantly dedicates her book to the untamed wild ones. I dedicate this foreword to all of us who long to know the fullness of the untamed, wild part of ourselves.

When I first encountered Jaiya's work, my partner, Peter, and I were beyond stuck. We were deeply in love but found ourselves to be completely sexually incompatible. We were frustrated, exhausted from trying and failing, and desperate to have the kind of sex we longed for. This was especially humiliating because I was busy teaching thousands and thousands of women about sex and sensuality. We took lots of different classes to find ways of connecting sexually, but nothing worked. Why?

We were completely missing the understanding of our Erotic Blueprints.

When the sex is not working, it sets in motion an avalanche of disapproval throughout the whole spectrum of the partnership. Peter was angry at me because he felt I did not love him enough. I was angry at Peter because I felt like he wasn't man enough in the bedroom, and I could not surrender to him.

What we did not realize at the time was that we had different Erotic Blueprints. We were unable to speak the other's language of pleasure, and after five years of this, the rift between us was so intense that we broke up.

As you'll soon discover in the pages of this book, there are five Blueprint Types. After finding Jaiya's work, I learned that my Primary Blueprint Type is the Sexual, which shed light on the disconnect between Peter and me. I was delivering huge workshops to thousands and thousands of women, and when I came offstage, I needed him to throw me down and fuck me so I could ground myself after holding all that energy. Peter, on the other hand, is wired primarily in the Energetic Blueprint. His body is so sensitive that I could literally breathe in his ear and he could go into full orgasm.

Jaiya's Blueprint methodology helped us bridge the chasm between our erotic styles. Finding a way to connect with each other has been one of the greatest adventures of my life, and I know he would say the same thing.

Once we each learned to speak the other's erotic language, a whole world of love and intimacy opened up for us. I am so grateful to Jaiya for giving us the knowledge and tools to find our way back to one another. Peter is the love of my life, and we now have a ridiculously hot and expansive sex life that just keeps getting better. We're able to speak all five of the Blueprints, which gives us access to endless worlds of exploration, connection, and deep love.

My wish for you, my little acorn? Use this book as your chance to grow.

Whatever your relationship status—single, partnered, multiple lovers—I want you to find your pathway to celebrate the fullness of the unique erotic being you are, and to communicate your truth to your lovers with joy and enthusiasm. This book gives you the tools to make it a reality.

this is a book about sexual awakening

This is an invitation. The words within these pages will take you into a sexual journey of deep self-realization. And through that awakening, a more fulfilling life awaits.

Fair warning: This path will lead you to places you haven't yet imagined.

So what does it mean to have a sexual awakening? You're about to find out.

There are many paths that lead us home to our true selves. Sexuality is only one path on this journey.

If you want to walk with me as your guide, I'm here. I don't come as a guru. I don't even come as a teacher these days. I come as a friend, a guide who can shine a light for you to find your own erotic intelligence, your own inner healer, your sexual home within.

First, allow me to introduce myself.

I've spent the past three decades working in the field of somatic sexology and have been at the forefront of a movement to destigmatize pleasure and sex. At the time of this writing, I've left a legacy of multiple books, online courses, and over three hundred coaches trained in the Erotic Blueprint Methodology. I've spent this lifetime dedicated to a mission to help end shame, pain, and confusion around sexuality. This book marks a new stage in my already amazing career. It's a departure for me, a journey into something deeper that I know in my soul will help expand the human experience. I'm honored every day that I get to hold others as they awaken to their deepest erotic selves.

Now let's talk about you.

This book is about you discovering who you are as an erotic being so that you can have a more fulfilling sexual life. But it goes much deeper than just sex. It's about your connection to yourself and to those you love. It's about awakening to who you actually are.

If you're single, this is the ideal time in your life to claim your erotic truth, without the needs and judgments of someone else telling you who you are or asking you to be someone you are not. This is your time to flower to full bloom, so when you encounter that next lover, you come skilled and ready to cultivate and experience passion and desire like you've never known before.

If you are in a relationship, this book is an opportunity to share your awakening with each other, so you can find nourishment, connection, fulfillment, and ultimate sexual satisfaction in the arms of your beloved(s).

Learning about sex is a lifelong adventure, and working within the Core Erotic Blueprints framework is a profound experience. It gets to the center of who you are and helps you free yourself. You'll be able to speak up about your desires and what you need to feel fulfilled.

This is not another sex technique book. I've written those books. I taught many a sex technique . . . and those are all fine and good for certain Erotic Blueprints. But honestly, my knowing hundreds of sex techniques was a very small contribution to having an incredibly hot and deeply connected sex life. More sex techniques will not get you there.

I hate to say it, being that I was a sex technique queen and still ended up in a near sexless relationship (which I'll share more about in chapter one). Yep, even sex experts struggle with getting the sex they really crave. Do you know why? It's because I was missing a key framework. I was missing the Erotic Blueprints!

The Erotic Blueprint framework is about acceptance and love of yourself and others, and eventually, it will help you become a master of something more profound than you've ever imagined.

Throughout this book, I'll share personal stories and the stories of people I've worked with. (Their names and details about their lives have been changed to protect their privacy. I have also combined some stories to further protect my clients and to drive a point home.) My clients are my biggest teachers. For that, I am eternally grateful. They've taught me about the struggles people go through on this journey to sexual awakening. They've taught me the power of love and perseverance. This book is the result of my many years of working with people seeking an amazing sexual life but finding themselves struggling to get there. It's also the result of working with people who aren't struggling but who know there is more to sex and want to experience all that is possible!

If you picked up this book, you may identify with one or more of the following statements, which I've heard from so many of my clients:

» "I struggle to find what turns me on and how to get what I want in the bedroom."

» "It feels like there is something more to sex that I just haven't been able to grasp, and I want the key to what's missing."

» "I feel like I'm the 'weird' one because I just don't fit into the mold of what society says I should be as an erotic being."

» "I feel broken and beyond all hope. I just know there's another level of fulfillment that has eluded me."

» "I'm in a relationship, and we love each other deeply, but when it comes to sex, it feels like we're a total mismatch."

» "I'm frustrated because it seems like my partner and I are just on different planets when it comes to sexual compatibility and desire."

» "I just don't know who I am, and I have a feeling that becoming better connected to my sexuality could help me learn more about myself."

» "I've taken so many personal growth workshops, yet none of them have worked. This is my last-ditch effort at a sexual awakening."

The Core Erotic Blueprints can help you solve many of these issues, and frankly, I've seen these Blueprints transform lives. After working with thousands of clients and seeing them go from extremely dissatisfied, feeling misunderstood and shut down, to sexually awakened and free to be who they are, I can say with confidence that knowing your Blueprint and how to express it, gaining the skills to master the turn-ons for all five Erotic Blueprint Types, and owning who you really are as an erotic being will change your life.

When we are awakened to who we truly are, we love ourselves enough to accept the gift of living a pleasure-filled life. And essentially, living a pleasure-filled life helps the world because we become happier human beings. (Don't get me started on orgasms and pleasure for world peace!)

This book is not meant to be a passive beach read—we're going to put things into practice! So take advantage of the Journaling Quickies, Embody It exercises, and—my favorite—Pleasure First experiences peppered throughout.

Are you ready to go on a sexual journey of a lifetime? Shall we begin?

CHAPTER ONE

how a sexologist ended up in a sexless relationship

Heaving sobs racked my curled-up body.

Yet another night rejected . . .

Feeling desperately alone . . .

And powerless to do anything about it.

How did it get to this?

How could I feel, just a year earlier, like I was a sex goddess on the top of my game, with a budding career as a world-renowned somatic sexologist, multiple lovers, and a hot, juicy sex life, but now feel like a fraud, convinced I couldn't get anyone to want to have sex with me, let alone the man I was deeply in love with?

How did this happen?

I mean, seriously—I knew all the sex techniques. I had even written a bestselling book on the topic, filled with techniques that I had personally mastered. I was an erotic massage pro, with over ten thousand hours of experience beneath my fingertips.

I felt beautiful. I was a confident businesswoman. And I knew how to please a lover.

So why couldn't I get Ian, my own partner, to have sex with me?

Why was I approaching him at night, ready and willing, desiring and offering sex, only to be told he was too tired, or wasn't interested? "Maybe tomorrow night?"

Why, when I wanted intercourse, was he approaching me with cuddles and hugs?

I started to wonder if maybe all the sex techniques, tips, and tools in the world wouldn't solve this issue. I just couldn't understand. I started to turn the rejection inward.

I was a new mom at the time, so maybe he didn't like my body anymore? Maybe having a baby together had tanked his libido? (Hint: Libido did play a role for sure.)

Maybe he just didn't love me anymore?

Maybe we weren't sexually compatible?

Maybe we weren't "meant" to be together?

I wasn't willing to give up. I set out on a journey to solve this challenge. A challenge I knew also plagued my clients.

The "best friends and roommates" scenario . . .

The dead bedroom . . .

The sexless marriage!

Maybe if I tried striptease? Would that turn him on?

Off I went to learn the art of erotic dancing.

I'll never forget coming home all excited to show him what I'd learned, to try out my "homework." I'm there in a G-string, with my butt in the air, in a sexy cat-pounce pose, and Ian says to me, "You don't need to do that, it's too obvious."

Ouch! I was crushed.

But I continued trying everything I could think of to get his sexual attention, to seduce him back into my arms and between my legs.

I thought maybe I wasn't being direct enough in showing him how much I desired him. I started doing things like touching his genitals while we were driving home from date night, or just flat-out saying, "I'd like to have sex tonight. Can we fuck?"

Most of my attempts fell flat, and conversations sometimes escalated into big arguments and tears. It all just seemed to make him uncomfortable. Little did I know that for Ian, my direct approach was more of a turn-off than a turn-on.

Nothing was changing. In fact, the emotional chasm between us was deepening, confusion and resentments were increasing, and the end of our loving relationship felt inevitable. We had tried it all. All the common advice available from internet searches, counselors, therapists, and sex educators.

And none of it worked!

Passion Is Not a One-Way Street

Ian was going through his own version of hell.

The economic crash of 2008 had devastated his once flourishing custom furniture design business. His confidence as a provider was at rock bottom. And the stress of raising our newborn son had tanked his libido. Because of a pelvic floor tear I had experienced while giving birth, sex had become painful for me, and Ian was scared to have sex with me because he didn't want to hurt me.

Yet there I was, still a force of sexual nature and erotic desire. My knowledge of the sexual arts, my level of erotic sensitivity, and my access to expanded states of consciousness sometimes left Ian feeling intimidated in the bedroom. He didn't have fifteen years of Tantric practice in his back pocket. Nor, at the time, did he have Sexological Bodywork training or other certifications and mastery of ancient erotic arts to rely on in our sex life.

While he loved me and was attracted to me, he couldn't figure out why he just didn't feel like having "on-demand" sex. He would come to bed to cuddle with me, hoping something intimate would unfold organically. Instead, he felt accosted by me going directly for his genitals and my desire for the certainty that we would have sex that night.

He wanted to connect and just let things unfold . . . very slowly.

I wanted certainty that we were going to have intercourse.

That need for certainty caused his desire to plummet and put pressure on him when he was already feeling so much external pressure.

So there I was, just wanting to go for it. I was approaching sex from what turned me on: "Let's have sex before the baby wakes up! Let's get to it and get to our orgasms. Let's play with each other naked with our hands and mouths all over each other."

And there he was, just wanting to slow things down, allow them to blossom and happen naturally, without any pressure or need for things to go a certain way. "Let's cuddle and hold each other and see what happens," he'd say. "Let's create space and delicious unfolding into one another. Let's explore and relax together." I'd roll my eyes at his poetic approach. It felt like we lived on two very different sexual planets. And I really couldn't understand his planet at all. Perhaps my sexpert ego had gotten the best of me.

What I couldn't see was that Ian was approaching sex from what turned him on. I was judging him based on his gender identification. *I mean, he's a man—he's supposed to want to have sex all the time! He's supposed to love blow jobs. What's wrong with him?*

17

The next few years certainly awakened me to the mythologies placed on cisgender men. I would also awaken to a revolutionary framework that would not only save my own sexual life, but completely transform the lives of my clients and the course of my career as well.

What I would discover from sitting in my own pain and my own sexless relationship turned out to be *the* thing that would go on to help millions of people around the world solve their "sexual incompatibility" divide and bridge this mismatch chasm. On our journey together, Ian and I unearthed a new language for erotic communication and sexual satisfaction that also empowered others to understand more deeply who they are as erotic beings, honoring their own unique sexuality and claiming more fully the pleasure that is the birthright of all human beings.

Claim the Pleasure You Deserve

I bet you're wondering what, exactly, I discovered.

Well, you're in luck! That's what the rest of this book is about.

I'm delighted to tell you that today, sixteen years later, Ian and I fall asleep with our limbs entwined, feeling unbelievably happy and content with our love life. We have an extraordinary sex life that really works for us.

Are there times when I still want more sex than he does? Of course! Does Ian still desire lots of space and time to allow sex to unfold organically? Absolutely! That's who we are as erotic beings. But we've both expanded to be able to speak the other's erotic language.

You see, the root of the issue was that Ian and I had different Erotic Blueprint Types (which I'll explain more in chapter three). Neither of us had the vocabulary to speak to the other about who we were sexually. Neither of us had developed the erotic language of the other.

On the surface, we were indeed totally mismatched. But both of us were willing to make the journey to expand into new sexual territory. We invested in the discovery of our own sovereign sexualities. As I developed this model to help us and the many clients I was serving, we learned the language of arousal and turn-on that would feed and fulfill our own passions and drive each other wild with desire once again. (Willingness, as you'll see, is a theme I return to later as an essential ingredient to creating the love and sex life you dream of having.)

That's when we began to see that we were wired differently in our eroticism. Owning our unique desires, capacities, and needs was an essential step on the path to cultivating deeply connected, passion-filled, and authentic intimacy.

To honor each other, we invested the time to stop speaking only the language of our own eroticism. We stopped relying on old habits in the bedroom, and instead began to learn each other's language. We met each other where we each desired to be met. We saw each other as we each wished to be seen.

And in that exploration . . .

Individually and together . . .

We experienced our sexual awakenings!

CHAPTER TWO

foundations for your erotic journey

Candace flipped her wrists over to show me the new tattoos she had etched onto her skin. "Because I always want to remember," she said, with excitement in her eyes.

Pleasure First

I looked at the beautifully scrolled letters and how strategically she had placed the words so that when she looked at her wrists, she could read them clearly. One of our core brand values had affected her life so much that she had venerated it with a tattoo. After always putting her own self-care and pleasure last, it was a life-affirming and transformational concept for Candace. It was a freeing and empowering act.

You know you're onto something when people are inspired to tattoo it on their bodies! Pleasure First is a foundational concept for our students and private clients.

The premise of Pleasure First is that we need delicious, yummy fuel to feed our lives. So many of us are running around like Candace on empty

Pleasure First: What Feels Good

During mindfulness practices, when we close our eyes and are asked to scan our body, our mind often chooses what is painful or uncomfortable. This practice is to help you notice what feels *good*.

Close your eyes. Take a couple of deep, slow breaths. Scan your body for what feels really good. Start at the bottoms of your feet. Work your way up your legs. Notice your genitals and pelvic floor. Don't forget your buttocks and anal area. Feel into your belly and lower back. Notice, with the rise and fall of your breath, what is pleasurable.

Move up into your chest, your upper back, and your shoulders. Notice your arms, neck, lips, face, and entire head. What feels lovely?

Now ask yourself this very important question: *How can this moment be even more pleasurable?*

Perhaps it's a shift in body position or adding more breath; maybe it's adding some touch, a stretch, or massage. Allow thoughts to percolate in your mind. Try whatever comes to you! Resist rushing from thing to thing, but really try any idea that might make your experience more pleasurable.

Continue this practice for as long as it feels good.

Your homework, or "homeplay," for the rest of the day is simply to ask yourself, *How can I make this moment even more pleasurable?*

tanks, expecting to be high-performance achievers. I used to be one of those high performers, trying to keep my tank optimized, but really running on fumes. Exhausted!

We live in a culture where we run, run, run around and then maybe, just maybe, achieve that next big goal and feel happy and fulfilled.

I now approach my life from the vantage of Pleasure First. What will truly fill my tank? What if I generate my own experience of happiness and find pleasure in the simplest of things? What if living life becomes pleasure itself? What practices could I do upon waking that would fuel my body and my eroticism from the day's very first breath?

I have found activating pleasure in my body, feeling truth through my body, to be one of the most powerful tools to creating the life I desire.

As you read this book you may think, *What in the world is Jaiya talking about?* That's okay. I'm often planting seeds that will sprout and bloom as you get closer and closer to your true erotic self. Stay on the path and keep practicing! Pleasure First is one of the primary ways in which we continue the practice.

I daresay that sexual awakening and spiritual awakening are very similar and lead to the same place. When referring to spirituality, the Sufis say, "The one who has tasted knows. The one who has not tasted will not know." You can tell a person about a food they've never tasted, but that description is nothing compared to actually tasting the food. At some level, talking about or describing sexual awakening falls flat; it can only be known from direct experience.

Think of it this way: Imagine you're trying to describe love to someone who has never had an experience of love. You can use a lot of words and a lot of metaphors, but they won't truly know what love is until they have the sublime experience of that extraordinary explosive orgasm of the heart.

So any time you feel like you don't understand or it seems like I'm contradicting or repeating myself, simply think, *This is Jaiya planting a seed, and when I have the direct experience of this, I'll know what she's talking about!*

This is not a prescriptive book. It's not a book about analyzing. It's a book where you arrive at truth in the moment.

I'll be continuously inviting you into the realm of experience. That realm includes a lot of discovery about your body. When you read words like "tune into your body" or "notice the effects" or "presence" or "embody," these are clues that you've received an invitation into direct experience.

"I'd rather learn from one bird how to sing than teach ten thousand stars not to dance," wrote revered poet E. E. Cummings. This is your time to not only learn to sing, but to sing, to dance, to fly, to orgasm your way into rapture! That is the realm of direct experience. At some point during this journey, you will know you've embodied these teachings because you'll be operating from a completely new baseline.

Sometimes I'll use metaphors to help plant seeds in your orgasmic garden. Sometimes poetry is the best way to describe that which is ineffable. When you see a metaphor or something feels like poetry, I'm pointing to a part of the process that can only be known through experience. I'm pointing you to yourself. In the famous words of Ram Dass, one of my favorite mentors, "We're all just walking each other home." And when you have the direct experience of these words, well, you'll realize that all there is to do is to serve and to be loved. So in essence, through the tool of sexual awakening, I, in service, am walking you home.

Sexy Foundations: Consent and Containers

Now that you're all juicy with noticing pleasure and have been given an invitation into direct experience, I'd like to offer you some other foundational guidelines for your journey before we dive into the Erotic Blueprints.

Like any good adventure, we need to make sure we have everything we need to make it the best possible experience.

This isn't a ride where I want you to keep your hands inside the cart at all times, or a situation where you always need to keep your hands to yourself. I want you to be free, and I want to make sure you stay as safe as possible. But like any game, there are certain rules that make it more enjoyable to play. Perhaps the idea of rules is a big turn-on for you, or maybe it makes you feel restricted and bound (and not in the good, kinky kind of way). If the idea of rules is challenging, think of this more as conscious foreplay that allows you to travel into higher and higher states of ecstatic pleasure.

CONSENT IS SEXY

Consent is about knowing what is a full-bodied "yes," what is a "maybe," what is a "willing to do," and what is a definite "hell no." With sexuality, it's vital that you have a conversation with your partner(s) about what you consent to and what you don't want in any experience. I want you to have the ability to find your full-bodied yeses and your strong nos so you don't end up regretting your experiences and contracting after you've expanded into new territory. A thwarted adventure is not an adventure at all. Sexual empowerment isn't just the freedom to say yes—it's also the freedom to have clear nos.

Before you do any of the exercises in this book, I advise you to have a consent conversation with a partner or friend. If you've been with your lover for many years, this conversation is especially important; we often have assumed consent in relationships, so it's a good practice to bring those assumptions out into the light and see if they really are true yeses or if something needs to shift.

And please understand that consent given can be taken away in an instant, at any time. And when someone's yes becomes a no, you must honor their no without hesitation.

Embody It: Full-Bodied Consent

STEP ONE: Think about a time when you were a "yes" to something. Something that you really wanted to do, but maybe were a little nervous about it. It doesn't have to be sexual; it could be anything, such as going to see a musician whose music you love. Close your eyes and imagine that thing that you really wanted to do. Now notice the sensations in your body that go along with what you are imagining. This is what it feels like when you are truly a yes to something.

STEP TWO: Think about a time when you were clearly a "no" to something. You really didn't want to do it—there was no question about it. Close your eyes and think about that thing. Notice the sensations in your body. Notice how this feels different from your yes.

Now you know what your yes and your no feel like! You can use this in the future when you're deciding whether something is a Fuck Yes or a Hell No.

What about when you are a "maybe"? Well, that's a time to pause. A maybe is a no in that moment with a possibility for a yes in the future, or with more information later down the path. Occasionally, a yes just takes time.

Remember: A yes can always become a no, but a no cannot become a yes.

Something may start as a no, but as things get heated up, we get drunk on all kinds of biochemicals. If we change our "sober" no to a yes in that moment, we often experience consent regret later, as the chemicals wear off. Consent regret is when we say yes to something in the moment but then regret it later. We want to avoid regretting saying yes in the heat of the moment, so if you're a no at the beginning of a play session, then that no is immutable. And if for any reason what you were a yes to becomes a no while you're playing, that must be honored.

The Power of Setting Your Container

Patty looked at me with absolute terror in her eyes and all over her body each time her lover mentioned that he wanted to go on some new wild sexual adventure. For five years, she'd been married to a man who craved what you might call the "extreme sports" end of the sexual spectrum. And he just wanted to take things further and further over the edge of experience.

Patty and her lover had never had a conscious consent conversation. And now she was holding on for dear life with no safety net and nothing that relaxed her enough for her own turn-on to blossom. Her body had started to shut down. She felt like she was free-falling, and he felt completely restricted in his erotic expression. Without clear boundaries for their sexual play, there was no safety for either of them, so they were stuck, completely frozen.

One of the most important things you can do when you're playing with any new sexual exploration is to create safety with a lot of conversations about what you each want to explore and what is off-limits. Patty and her husband had never done this, and it was destroying their intimacy.

Consent is one part of a bigger conversation around creating a "container of safety" for your lover. Think of a container as something that holds your experience. Without the container, we don't know what the boundaries of the experience are; there is a lack of safety, and the environment isn't one in which we can comfortably play. Containers help us play all the way to our edges. Edges are the borders for our erotic play and exploration. We don't want to go past the edge, but to play right up to it.

The container of safety is one of the first things I teach any of my clients.

Safety is often missed as a foundational element to experiencing orgasmic pleasure and sexual satisfaction. To me, it is one of the sexiest parts of making love. Safety can be a huge turn-on. Safety creates the possibility for surrender to pleasure and the freedom to fully explore, within the bounds of the agreed-upon container.

My clients occasionally have a little resistance to the container of safety (Patty's husband certainly did), but once they get the hang of it, they end up creating very sexy containers in which to play.

For example, over dinner, simply share the answers to these three questions with your lover:

» "What would you like to explore tonight in bed?" (Desires)
» "What are your boundaries for tonight?" (Consent Conversation)
» "What is the signal that I need to pause or stop if something feels like too much?" (Safety Measures)
» "What kind of environment will help you feel most open to pleasure?" (Space Setting)

Creating a container is so important for certain Blueprint Types. Without a container, they can feel ungrounded, unsafe, and unsure—which isn't sexy for them at all. So be sure that you create a strong, safe container in which you've discussed erotic consent (your individual yeses and nos). Taking this time to create a container of safety before you make love will lead to a world of difference in the level of arousal and pleasure you experience.

This also goes for emotional safety as you're practicing the exercises in this book. One powerful agreement you can make with your partner before you begin is that you'll give each other the freedom to be completely

Embody It: A Safety Dyad

For this exercise, you will need a friend to share with or a journal to write in. Set a timer for twenty minutes and answer this prompt over and over until the timer goes off.

Prompt: "Tell me something that would help you feel safe during sex."

If you need some inspiration, here are some responses from Bradley, one of my clients:

» To tell the person I'm with that I'm sensitive and need to go slow.

» To know that my "no" will be honored and not overridden.

» To know that we won't have penetration at all, or until I'm ready for it.

» To hear "I love you" from the person I'm with.

» To have the doors locked and the windows closed.

» To be in a private space without any interruptions or loud noises.

» To go really, really slow.

» To feel that I can stop at any time and not be pressured further.

I encourage you to find your own responses and to practice this exercise with your lover or a friend as a way to communicate what will make you feel safest in that moment.

Some of my clients, like Bradley, eventually learn to do these dyad exercises as part of their foreplay before they make love—this can leave you feeling safer, heard, and ready to play!

honest. For example, you may say, "Your desires are safe with me"—but only say it if you mean it! If your partner opens up to you and you punish them for their honesty and free expression, that's not cool.

Remember that just because your lover shares a desire doesn't mean you are obligated to fulfill that desire for them. You always have the freedom to find where your desires intersect—that's consent. And consent is sexy.

Fulfilling sexual connection and mind-blowing sexual satisfaction are achieved on a foundation of safety. It's an essential ingredient when it comes to experiencing your full erotic potential. Learning to establish safety for every Blueprint Type, therefore, is a must.

Physical safety, emotional safety—safety always comes first.

Becoming skilled in setting up containers of safety, where boundaries are clear and honored and consent for any and all activities has been clearly given, is a requirement for those who wish to explore sex in a healthy way.

Pleasure first—check!

Consent conversations—check!

Container setting—CHECK!

Safety—CHECK! CHECK!

I believe we're ready to turn on the ignition of our eroticism and go exploring! In the next chapter, I'm going to introduce to you the Core Erotic Blueprints, and we'll take the next step on our quest for erotic self-realization. I'm so thrilled to be your guide as you uncover deeper truths about your sexuality and start living from those truths, ultimately creating more pleasure, love, and well-being for yourself and other people. You've just begun the journey of a lifetime.

CHAPTER THREE

who are we?
erotic blueprints
are born

As I watched him shaking and gyrating in orgasmic delight, his eyes wide, it hit me.

"What's happening?" he exclaimed.

"You're wired energetically," I said.

His wife continued to hover her hands over his body as the volume on his turn-on rose higher and higher. At that moment, after all the years of training, working with my clients, and leading Tantra workshops and group sessions, the words of my mentors all came into focus and . . .

The Erotic Blueprints were born.

Like any birth, every idea has a gestation time, and I had gestated this one for many years. I'm certain it wasn't any one specific thing, but instead many influences over many years of helping people have erotic breakthroughs and experience lasting transformation. And as you learned in chapter one, I was seeking to resolve major challenges in my own love life, and the Blueprints were a relationship-saver.

Your Core Erotic Blueprint is the key to unlocking a treasure trove of hidden pleasures, just waiting for you to claim them. Sometimes on this journey it feels more like you're remembering something long forgotten than discovering something new. Deep down, we all truly know how to love ourselves and each other; sometimes, we just need to be reminded.

Are you ready to remember?

Who Are We as Erotic Beings?

I've always loved personality-type tests like Myers-Briggs and the DiSC profile because they've helped me understand more about myself and validated how I thought, behaved, and interacted with others in the world. I've received great insights from different tests, which have allowed me to see myself in a deeper light.

Could there be a similar typing for our erotic selves?

What makes one person more introverted and another feel energized from partying all night long with friends? Why does one person shine as a leader while another thrives working behind the scenes? Why is one person turned on by being tied up and bound and another turned on from not being touched at all? Who are we? Who am *I*?

I was just eighteen when I set out to answer that question.

In 2006, during my training as a somatic sexologist, I met Jack Morin, author of *The Erotic Mind*. In meeting him, something came together in my mind.

In his book and teachings, he spoke of something called the Core Erotic Theme. What I loved about uncovering a Core Erotic Theme was that it wasn't based on dysfunction. Instead, Jack mapped a person's eroticism based on "peak erotic experiences." A peak erotic experience is something

Pleasure First: Erotic Tools

Let's experiment with some erotic tools: breath, movement, sound, touch, and visualization.

Close your eyes. Scan your body for what feels good and pleasurable, all the way from your toes to the top of your head. What feels alive and delicious?

Now choose one area that feels amazing; if you can't find an area that feels amazing, choose a place that feels good or neutral. Put your attention on that area. Just notice what comes up as you put your attention there. There's no need to change anything—just give it your attention.

Now add **breath**. Take a deep breath into the area where you're putting your attention. Exhale slowly through your mouth and then inhale again through your nose. Continue to put your attention on this area and notice what happens when you add breath. Does it intensify pleasure, or does it take away pleasure? Simply notice without judgment. It's all just information.

Now add **sound**. As you breathe in through your nose, simply relax your awareness of this area. As you exhale, you can make the sound of how this spot on your body feels; perhaps it's a sigh, or a moan, or a gentle hum. Just notice what comes up as you make gentle sounds. If making a sound feels uncomfortable, again, just notice the area.

Let's try some **movement**. Place your attention on this resourced area, which is any area on your body where you are experiencing pleasure. What happens if you add some gentle movement? Maybe you stretch or rotate your joints. Experiment with different movements to find what feels most pleasurable, and don't forget that perhaps stillness is what is most pleasurable.

How about **touch**? What happens when you place a hand on this area you've been working with? Or you could add some massage? Notice what happens and what you become aware of as you add touch. Does it increase or decrease pleasure?

And finally, let's add some **visualization**. What's a pleasurable thing for you to imagine? Perhaps making love with someone you desire? Maybe a steamy scene with a lover or spouse? What can you visualize that may turn you on? Notice what happens as you put your attention on this area while you add a hot visualization.

Now come back to the area you started with. Notice the effects of the practice on this area and then bring your awareness to the rest of your body. Take a moment to journal how using these erotic tools affected you.

that stands out as an unforgettably wonderful experience. By uncovering an individual's peak experiences, Jack could see a theme emerge regarding what turned that person on and how it tied to their overall sexual expression. This was their Core Erotic Theme.

I thought back to the 1990s, when I was studying Tantra. In a workshop, we were asked to share with another workshop participant three of our most extraordinary erotic experiences; then the person with whom we shared would tell us if they noticed any theme reflected within those three experiences. One of the peak experiences I shared was about one of my lovers who knew I had a fantasy of being a courtesan, so he had decorated our bedroom with exotic fabrics and plates of dates and mangoes, and set up a plan where for twenty-four hours, he would be different men coming to experience a few hours with a courtesan (costume changes were included). Twenty years later, the encounter still stands out as a highlight in my sexual life.

This curiosity about who I was erotically and what themes showed up again and again led me to desire to know others in the same way. I discovered that I was a person who was turned on by blowing someone's mind erotically, rocking their world with epic sexual adventures that they had always wanted but had never allowed themselves. I was so fascinated by this process that I spent the next decade paying attention to themes in the many stories of peak erotic experiences relayed to me by clients and others.

Just a few years later, I had the opportunity to be mentored by Joseph Kramer, who created an entire profession—Sexological Bodywork—around educating people about their bodies and how to use that knowledge to find and embrace their erotic selves. While I had had years of learning about quality touch as a massage therapist—in which the erotic was always forbidden—this was an entirely new way to be with the body. It felt whole.

This specialized licensure allowed us to teach people about anatomy, about touch, and about pleasure. It wasn't just talking about sex—it was about embodying sex!

Journal Quickie:
Exploring Peak Experiences

Take out a journal or find a close friend to share with.

Write down or share three of your peak erotic experiences.

As you write, notice the things that turned you on the most. Notice what about each encounter made it a peak experience. Notice what happens in your body as you write down or recall the experience.

If you feel you have not had a peak erotic experience, you can include close intimate experiences with yourself or with others that felt positive to you. (Not everyone has had a peak erotic experience; hopefully this book will lead you to one!)

If you are doing this exercise with a friend, have them give you a reflection of what stood out to them thematically.

If you are writing in a journal, read through your experiences and notice if there are any similarities among them. What themes made these experiences so great for you?

Joseph's work was a major influence on me in so many ways, from inquiring about all that was erotically possible in our bodies to learning how to be present with another person through touch and mapping how pleasure worked in their body. Joseph taught me how to help someone create a pleasure map of their body, something you'll be learning more about in chapter twelve.

In 2009, I met the brilliant Esther Perel. She had studied with Jack Morin herself, so the two of us had instant rapport. In her book *Mating in Captivity*, she devotes an entire chapter to the idea of Erotic Blueprints.

Embody It: Erotic Inquiry

Satyen Raja, creator of WarriorSage and the Accelerated Evolution Academy, taught me the importance of going back and forth between two polarities during erotic inquiry. The name of this inquiry exercise is kenshō, which means "seeing one's true nature."

Do this exercise with a partner or friend who can give you their full attention or write it out in a journal. Start by deciding who will be person A and who will be person B, then set a timer for forty minutes.

Person A will prompt person B: "Feel who you are as an erotic being."

Person B will feel that and notice what comes up as they contemplate who they are for at least twenty seconds and then report what arose from that contemplation.

Person A says "thank you" to signify that they understand. It is important that this practice is about understanding, not agreeing with what feels true or isn't true.

Person A again prompts person B: "Feel who you are *not* as an erotic being."

Person B will now feel something or someone they are not erotically. It is important that they focus on and contemplate something or someone specific. For example, if you feel you are *not* George Washington, feel what it is to be George Washington, and then share what came up as you contemplated this. Notice body sensations, thoughts, emotions, and images that arise. Do this for at least twenty seconds and then share what comes up with your partner.

Remember that you are not reporting about the thing or person you focused on but instead on what came up as you were contemplating that person or thing.

For example, you wouldn't say, "I'm not Sally—a person who is shut down." You might say, "What came up is a cold feeling, a tense, shut-off feeling."

Person A will say "thank you" to signify that they understand.

Now switch roles and repeat the exercise.

Keep working alternating roles like this until the forty minutes are up. Don't allow yourself to get into a conversation about what you are sharing; simply go back and forth, inquiring and reporting.

After forty minutes, share with each other or journal about who you are as an erotic being.

"Tell me how you were loved," she says, "and I'll show you how you make love." This brought to mind a question: Is our eroticism shaped by our upbringing?

From my work over the past twenty-five years, I would say the answer is: absolutely.

Who are we without the conditioning and programming of our early upbringing? Who are we without our coming-of-age embarrassments, shame, and traumas? How did our parents, religious affiliation, or hometown shape what turns us on today? Or were we born this way? Or is it a little of both?

And the Erotic Blueprint Types Were Born

I was in my office working with the couple I spoke of earlier in this chapter. He was having a lot of difficulty feeling turned on and achieving an erection. I had him lie on the massage table with his eyes closed, and I began to do a body-mapping session on him.

I started by showing his wife how to hover her hands over him, not touching him physically but feeling him energetically.

Then it happened . . .

His eyes opened wide and he looked at me with shock. "What's happening?" he asked.

As his wife hovered her hands above him, he got an erection and his body started quivering. He was shocked. She was shocked. All this time his eroticism wasn't in all the sexual techniques they'd tried—it was in him having space, in the teasing, and in the energetic play off his body!

In that moment, everything—my fifteen years of studying and mastering somatic exploration, Tantra, and the ancient erotic arts, plus the wisdom of my mentors and the work I had done with hundreds of clients—crystallized into a clear framework and language for erotic communication.

That day I journaled with a deep thrill and knowing about the first three Blueprint Types: Energetic, Sensual, and Sexual: *It seems that people ARE wired differently. There are three different types or Blueprints so far. I'm seeing people who are Energetically Wired, or turned on by not being touched . . .*

Over the next few months, as I paid more and more attention to how people's bodies responded to different touches, the Kinky and Shapeshifter Blueprints revealed themselves. And over the next five years, I utilized my clinical experience and my work with clients, as well as my personal experience healing the painful abyss between my partner Ian and me, to create the entire system of the Core Erotic Blueprints.

A Glimpse of the Five Erotic Blueprint Types

An **ENERGETIC** is most turned on by anticipation, space, tease, and longing.

A **SENSUAL** can be deeply embodied and is most turned on by having all their senses ignited.

A **SEXUAL** is turned on by what we think of as "sex" in our culture: nudity, penetration, orgasms, and lots of intercourse.

A **KINKY** is turned on by and eroticizes the taboo.

A **SHAPESHIFTER** is turned on by all of it, loves it all, and wants more.

It was exhilarating to finally find an erotic language, and a way to meet people's sexual needs.

I started to get feedback from my clients like "I'm not broken after all." Or "We finally have a way to talk about who we are erotically." Or "Now everything makes sense." And, of course, my personal sex life underwent a massive transformation as Ian and I discovered we were very different types: he was Sensual/Kinky, and I was Sexual/Energetic.

Five years after discovering the Erotic Blueprints and testing their effectiveness with clients and in my own bedroom, I was confident in their validity and ready to take them out into the world. As I began sharing publicly, I found, to my great surprise, that most people resonated immediately with these ideas.

I wanted to make sure the framework held up. And it did—in 2016, we launched the Erotic Blueprint Quiz and Erotic Blueprint Breakthrough Course to educate people on this comprehensive system for sexual wellness and erotic satisfaction.

Understanding who we are and what turns us on is just one step on the path to erotic self-realization. We also need to see where we have been and what has influenced us erotically, and become cognizant of and reshape our existing thoughts and feelings about sex and eroticism.

If we're going to build a mansion of otherworldly pleasures together, we can't start on a broken foundation and expect it to stand.

But most of us *have* built our erotic life on a cracked and crumbling foundation. We've cobbled together our concepts of sex and pleasure from inherited and disempowering beliefs; embodied shame; faulty assumptions; bad sex education; traumatic experiences; and learning from peers, porn, and propaganda. Before we can reconstruct a new, vital, and orgasmic sex life, we need to take a wrecking ball to the decrepit old structure that no longer serves us as the erotic beings we have become.

We need to bust some myths.

CHAPTER FOUR

erotic myths

If you picked up this book, you're probably trying to gain a greater understanding of sex, so where, exactly, can you find the truth? Is what a scientific study says the truth? Is it what our religious upbringing told us? How about what Mom, Dad, or Grandma taught us about sex? Is it what your friends told you through giggles, blushes, or brags? Or is it what you learned from watching porn or romantic comedies or read in the latest mainstream magazine? Or is it something found in your personal past experiences?

In this book, I'm going to continually point you back to this idea of inquiry for yourself. I'm going to guide you to your own truth. No more looking outside yourself for the answers. We're going to go in. And we're especially going to go into your body. We are going to go into the soul of sex. Let go of everything you thought you knew. We're going to expand your definitions of sex and pleasure and what it means to have a sexually fulfilling relationship with yourself.

Remember: I'm not the guru here—you are. Your body is. Your pleasure is your guide.

It's time for you to come home to what is true for *you*. And that right there is sexual empowerment—that is healthy and whole sexuality.

When it comes to sex, the world abounds with mythologies, assumptions, and cultural norms. I love to stick a pin in these. Let's get closer to your sexual truth by looking at some significant myths that I regularly hear clients have bought into.

Myth #1: Something Must Be Wrong with You If . . .

So many messages out there give you the opportunity to feel bad about yourself.

Something must be wrong with you if you aren't having mind-blowing, earthshaking, scream-inducing orgasms. Something must be wrong with you if your body doesn't look a certain way. Something must be wrong with you if you're older or if you're a person with a disability. Something must be wrong with you if you don't fit the cultural norm. Something must be wrong with you if your genitals don't look like someone else's. Something must be wrong with you if you don't identify with the genitals you were born with. Something must be wrong with you if you love more than one person or step outside the conventional narratives of love and sexuality.

These harsh judgments are just the tip of the "what's wrong with me" iceberg.

Inadequate sex education, combined with over a century of sexuality research focused primarily on dysfunction, has created a lot of unnecessary suffering in our sex lives. A lot of what we know about sex today doesn't consider gender, orientation, culture, or stage of life. It can be easy to diagnose ourselves as "not normal" when we view ourselves in the restrictive context of the values and attitudes we've inherited around sex. There is no clear understanding of what "normal" is—because normal doesn't exist. In a relationship, these ideas about what is normal can become amplified because of our differing ideas about sex.

No wonder so many of us are hung up on and confused about sex!

The world loves to reflect to you how much there is wrong with you. And even if you try to follow the "right" path, there's always an opposing view out there somewhere.

But what if, in fact, there's nothing wrong with you at all?

What if your body—its shape, its size, its ability—is perfect? What if you are whole and complete just the way you are? What if no one is broken? What if your genitals are absolutely lovely (and normal, I might add—diversity is the norm!), even if someone, somewhere, told you they weren't? Creating your personal Erotic Blueprint map (which we'll do in chapter fifteen) will help you realize you are not broken.

In interviews, when I'm asked if I have a final message for listeners, readers, or viewers, I frequently respond that if people take one thing away from the interview, it would be this: You are not broken, and you never were. You are whole and complete just the way you are. You do not need anyone outside yourself to validate you. You loving you is the point of this game.

We live in a sexually Blueprinted culture. How many TV shows and movies have you seen where sex means intercourse between a heterosexual cisgender man and a heterosexual cisgender woman? This leads many of us to think that if we don't fit inside that sexual narrative, something must be wrong with us. But most of us have an erotic wiring that differs from that "standard" cultural norm.

There is no one way to be based on your gender, your age, your body type, or anything else. You are you, and you are wired in your own unique way.

You can only be you.

Myth #2: The Problems in Your Sex Life Are Because of Incompatibility

I want you to imagine for a moment that you've fallen in love with the person of your dreams. This person is deeply in love with you. Everything feels amazing, and you know you want to be in a relationship with them.

Now imagine that they speak French and you speak English. Would you end the relationship because you speak different languages?

No.

Would you learn each other's languages because you're in love with that person and want to make the relationship work?

Yes.

I don't believe in sexual incompatibility, and here's why: In my almost three decades of working with people who believe they have a sexual "mismatch" of sorts, I've discovered it's not about partners being on different pages—it really comes down to three things:

1. YOU DO NOT KNOW WHO YOU ARE AND WHAT TURNS YOU ON EROTICALLY.

How can you expect your lover to pleasure you if you don't actually know what you want or like? If you let others tell you who you are or who you are supposed to be, and you haven't discovered your unique form of sexual expression, you will end up unsatisfied after most erotic encounters. You've bought into the myth that something is wrong with you.

2. YOU ARE NOT COMMUNICATING HONESTLY ABOUT SEX.

If you expect your partner to read your mind and know exactly what to do to please you, you're in for infinite disappointment. So many people don't know how to communicate about sex, or feel so much shame around owning their desires that they hide out in the dark, wondering why their sex life is so confusing, frustrating, and dissatisfying.

I see it so often. Lovers are not sexually incompatible. Rather, they have never learned a language to communicate their sexual needs and desires. They have never talked about what they want to try together. What is true for most people is that our lovers want to please us, to bring us satisfaction. Lack of erotic self-awareness, of a language to communicate needs and desires, and of open and honest communication are the biggest reasons things don't work out sexually for people who love each other.

In the field of sexology, sexual incompatibility is known as sexual desire discrepancy (SDD). SDD is seen as a complex and multifaceted issue, and it typically gets attributed to the person with lower sexual desire. Problems with low sexual desire or SDD are some of the most common causes of distress in relationships, and are the primary reason couples go to see a sex therapist. While considerable attention is focused on why people show minimal interest in sex, the context in which sex is desired or unwanted is ignored.

Canadian clinical psychologist and sexologist Peggy J. Kleinplatz has spent decades investigating what makes up "optimal sexual experiences." Her research team consistently identified eight components of optimal sexual experiences, regardless of gender or sexual orientation: being utterly embodied, being in synch, deep erotic intimacy, authenticity, high levels of communication (verbal and touch), interpersonal risk-taking, vulnerability, and transcendence.

Embody It: Opening Communication with Your Partner

The biggest hurdle to communicating about sex is often our fear of losing love or hurting a partner's feelings. We don't want to make anyone feel bad, or as if they've done something wrong. Here's a simple approach to beginning the conversation.

Say something positive: Start by mentioning something your partner does that you like, especially something that relates to what you wish to discuss with them.

Example: "I love how you touch me and how willing you are to please me."

Create a safe, raw, and real space: Start by sharing your own vulnerability about the topic and then explain directly that they have done nothing wrong. Be open to hearing and doing what would create more safety for them, and be open to sharing what would create safety for you.

Example: "I love our intimacy and I want us to keep exploring how we can have even more pleasure in our sex life together. I feel scared to talk to you about sex, because sex was something that felt shameful to talk about growing up. I want you to know that this is scary for me, that you haven't done anything wrong, and I wonder what would create a safe space for you to talk with me about our sex life."

Make a request: Convey to your partner that you are making a request, not placing a demand on them. Do not expect that your lover will want to talk about the subject, and don't act combative if they're resistant to having the conversation.

Example: "I'm curious if you would like to talk about this now, or if you'd like to have dinner with me on Friday and we can talk about it then. Or is there a time that works better for you?"
You have now opened the door for the conversation!

3. YOU ARE UNWILLING TO LEARN THE SKILLS TO PLEASE YOUR LOVER.

If you're unwilling to master the skills to please your lover (or vice versa), then I'm sorry to tell you that your journey together ends there.

Reluctance to explore intimacy with your partner is often the biggest reason for a failing sex life. That's not incompatibility—it's an unwillingness to do what it takes to learn your lover's erotic language. It's that you don't know who you are erotically and what turns you on, you haven't learned or have been unwilling to learn the skills to please your partner, or you and your partner have been speaking different erotic languages and didn't know it. But if you're open-minded, anything is possible! It really does come down to learning the skills.

Myth #3: All Cisgender Men Are Sexual and Dominant, and All Cisgender Women Are Sensual and Submissive

Whether or not we're aware of it, we've been receiving cultural messages about gender-appropriate ways to behave since birth. This impacts how we operate in the world and also influences our sexual behaviors. While there is no research to support the stereotypes that cisgender men (a person who identifies with their sex *assumed* at birth, meaning if they're gendered male as a boy, they identify as being a male in adulthood) are the Sexual Blueprint and cisgender women are the Sensual Blueprint, most people are conditioned to have certain sexual desires and behaviors.

In their 1973 book *Sexual Conduct*, sociologists John Gagnon and William Simon first introduced sexual script theory as a framework for understanding sexual interactions and scenarios. They theorized that sexual scripts are shaped by gender roles, sexual roles, and relationship norms. They start out as cultural scripts that become our interpersonal scripts, which then over time become our pattern. Sexual scripts influence gendered stereotypes in the bedroom. These heteronormative scripts are generally characterized by gendered power inequality (men are sexually dominant and women are sexually submissive). This creates obstacles and is sometimes harmful when we try to expand what is erotically possible beyond the scripts we've been given.

Research also suggests a sexual double standard that judges women harshly for being more sexually assertive or engaging in "casual sex," while a man's masculinity may come under attack if he isn't sexually assertive enough. The pressure to stay within our assigned gendered sexual roles limits how we believe we can experience sexual pleasure, especially if we don't want to be rejected by a partner.

In my own life, I was guilty of projecting this mythology onto Ian. I had an expectation that Ian's sexuality should be expressed by wanting tons of intercourse and oral sex. Luckily, I came to learn how wrong this projection was, and how to honor him in the ways he wanted to be loved.

Over two million people have taken our quiz, and we've seen that the gendered definitions of what it means to be a "man" or a "woman" aren't serving anyone. From analyzing data from the quiz, we've found that cisgender men are not Sexual across the board. Men can—and do—express and experience sexual fulfillment in many ways (some of which are viewed as not stereotypically masculine). Any time we box someone of any gender into one way of being, we may be doing an injustice to their optimal experience of connection and pleasure. So let's please stop reinforcing the myth that all men just want sex and that their sexuality is easy and simple.

It simply isn't true.

We also discovered that when it came to heterosexual cisgender women, most were the Energetic Blueprint Type (you'll learn more about what this means in the next chapter). The Sensual Blueprint came up as the second most self-identified type. But many women also identify with the Kinky, Sexual, and Shapeshifter Types.

All of this to say, we can't put sexuality in a box based on the genitals someone was born with, the gender they were assigned at birth, or the gender they identify as now. We are each our own unique erotic being, and no one way is the "right way" for any gender to express arousal and turn-ons.

Myth #4: Something Must Be Wrong If You Are Seeking Out Sex Advice

There is so much stigma when it comes to getting sex advice. Once when a celebrity client of mine was a guest on a popular daytime talk show, I watched in horror as the hosts made fun of her for openly discussing getting sex advice and learning about her Erotic Blueprint. They expressed that if she needed sex advice two years into her relationship, the relationship must be doomed.

I couldn't believe she was being shamed for getting help with her sex life!

We don't shame people for wanting help to learn how to manage their money, master a sport, or play a musical instrument. We don't shame people for talking about the great tennis coach they had or the great teacher who inspired them. We don't shame people for seeing a therapist or hiring a life coach. But there it was: shaming someone for seeking help with sexuality—something most of us don't get properly educated on anyway—and for talking about it so openly.

So let me just set the record straight. Smart people know that having mentors and learning about any topic they find important is invaluable.

That's why you're reading this book.

There is nothing wrong with seeking help, and no, you are not doomed if you talk with other people about what you're learning and what's going on with your sex life. If you have this book in your hands, if you are learning about your sexuality, if you are taking the Erotic Blueprint Breakthrough Course, if you've hired a coach or mentor in this area—YOU ARE BRILLIANT.

You're intelligently and consciously learning something new!

Myth #5: Sex Tricks and Techniques Will Solve It All

You read my personal story in chapter one—I was a "Sex Goddess" who had written books filled with amazing sex techniques, yet there I was, leading an unfulfilling, sexless existence.

Knowing tricks and techniques is great. But it didn't help me. And no matter how many technique-based skills I gave my clients, it wasn't helping them, either. If you use a great technique designed to please a Sexual Blueprint on an Energetic Type, you'll see their arousal drop like a stone. Use an Energetic Practice with a Sexual Type, and not only will the Sexual's turn-on go limp, they may also look at you like you've got three heads. "What the hell are you doing?"

In my work trying to solve the issues my clients and I were facing, I realized teaching them another sex technique wasn't going to solve their core challenges. There was so much more going on. There was so much healing that needed to happen, and frankly, most of the techniques out there are designed for Sexuals and don't work for everyone else.

The Erotic Blueprints empower you to "Blueprintify" your pleasure, giving you practices, tools, and techniques designed to thrill and fulfill the intimate cravings of *all* the Blueprint Types. With Blueprintified techniques, you increase your erotic intelligence, understand your unique turn-on map, and know exactly how to navigate the erogenous terrain of your lover's body. With Blueprintified touch skills—a delicate teasing stroke here, a nibble right there—you become the erotic artist, deeply connected and penetrating, able to deftly inspire your lover's arousal and orgasmic delight. You can confidently ride endless waves of pleasure. And when you expand into appreciating the pleasures of all the Erotic Blueprint Types, you will discover how to Blueprintify any sex technique—that's erotic mastery. You'll learn just how to do this later in this book.

Myth #6: Sex Is Just Physical

Definitely not. This ties into our limited definition of sex and our limited idea of what sex is supposed to be. Sex most often involves bodily contact—but not all the time.

One of the topics that spurred a viral discussion on the internet was the "touchless" orgasm that my partner Ian demonstrated with me during episode two of *Sex, Love & Goop* on Netflix. In the scene, I'm blindfolded, and Ian is hovering his hands over my body. Without me seeing him or being touched, I'm writhing around on the massage table in orgasmic bliss. If you've seen the episode . . .

Yes, I did have an orgasm.

No, I wasn't faking it.

The idea that sex is just physical and that you should be having mind-blowing orgasms and pleasure from intercourse or from rubbing your clitoral head vigorously or from the latest oral sex technique just leaves most people feeling broken, wrong, and hopeless. But there are so many amazing possibilities in the energetic realms, and there's a whole Erotic Blueprint that operates in this zone of pleasure most of the time.

And wouldn't you agree that sex is also emotional? Have you ever cried after a great orgasm? Or felt deep love and connection to yourself or another human being? Have you ever felt joy and ecstasy during lovemaking? Or had angry makeup sex? Sex without emotion is like a movie without a musical score (try watching a movie on mute—it's not very exciting).

The first step to broadening your definition of sex is to open your mind and body to all that it can be.

Myth #7: Your Sexuality Is Fixed

In 2015, Dr. Sari van Anders, a neuroscientist, award-winning researcher, and fellow of the American Psychological Association, published a comprehensive framework about a person's sexual fluidity called sexual configurations theory (SCT). Based on years of sex and gender research, SCT challenged the ideas that gender is binary and that sexual attraction is only based on gender. Rather, sexual desire is influenced by people's lived experiences and includes an entire range of gender and sexual diversity, not just what the culture deems as "normal."

What I have seen repeatedly during the almost thirty years of my career is that we all can get caught up in feeling like we have a fixed identity when it comes to sex, our preferences, and our ideas of who we are.

This greatly limits us.

When we get fixed in our identity and our story about that identity, we stop growing; we close ourselves off to the infinite orgasmic possibilities that surround us. We become inflexible, and lack creativity when confronted with the inevitable changes that wisdom and aging bring to our sexuality. It's okay to get stuck. And it's okay to want to defend your identity, especially if you fought hard for it.

Remember: You aren't broken. ("Broken" is a self-identity that frequently shows up in sexuality.) And we can't bypass the parts of ourselves that get trapped in fixed identities ("I'm a broken person," "I'm a prudish person," "I'm a slutty person"). They have a goal or a desire that hasn't been met yet. That desire might be for more safety, for understanding and acceptance, for love and connection.

I've seen firsthand how identity shifts, how life itself transforms, how we are much more fluid in our turn-ons than we previously thought ourselves to be.

Think about it: Are you the same person you were at five years old? Do you have the same body? Is your sexuality the same as it was when you were a teenager? If you are a parent, how did having a child affect your sexuality? If you are going through menopause, what is happening to your sexuality as you enter this new phase of life?

I teach clients how to reclaim parts of themselves by helping them reintegrate those fixed identities, so that they have the freedom to step into new ones.

The results are profound.

Someone who said they hated sex in the morning suddenly loves it.

Someone who said they just didn't like sex at all suddenly can't get enough.

Someone who lived in shame and shut down around their turn-ons opens to their kinky side and delights in their newfound freedom and consensual fun.

Someone who behaved like a Sexual their entire life realizes that they are really sensitive and Energetic.

Someone who said they were heterosexual fell in love with someone of the same sex.

Embody It: The Relationship-Evolving Dyad

I learned this exercise in my early days of teaching Tantra and through the guidance of my mentor Satyen Raja. The exercise allows you to become present with a partner and go deeper than you would in a normal conversation.

In fact, this isn't conversation—it's communication.

During this exercise, you or your partner may share things that are deeply surprising, previously unknown, and even triggering. Remember, you are not seeking to agree with anything they say. You are seeking deeper authenticity and *understanding* about yourself and your partner. (If you are not in a relationship, you can do this exercise with yourself in a journal.)

Begin by deciding who will be person A and who will be person B. Then put your loving attention on each other, giving each other your full presence. Do this for one to two minutes, then begin.

For each of the three prompts, person A will prompt person B, and person B will respond.

If person A understands what person B has shared, they respond with "Thank you." If they do not understand, they can respond with "Clarify that," "Say it again," or "Summarize that."

Person B can respond until person A has a full understanding.

Switch. Continue going back and forth for ten minutes, then move on to the next prompt.

PROMPT ONE: "TELL ME SOMETHING YOU LOVE ABOUT ME."
This prompt creates a connection between you.

PROMPT TWO: "TELL ME SOMETHING YOU WANT ME TO UNDERSTAND ABOUT YOU."

This prompt helps you understand each other. You can make the prompt more specific if you're dealing with a charged emotion about a particular topic. For example, "Tell me something you want me to understand about you and sex."

PROMPT THREE: "TELL ME SOMETHING YOU THINK WE AGREE UPON."

This prompt creates a shared reality between you. You can also make it specific to something you are working on together. For example, "Tell me something you think we agree upon about sex." Remember that you don't have to agree.

At the end of this exercise, you may want to again share things that you love about each other, or simply hug, kiss, or cuddle to feel the connection.

Someone who said they are broken realized they're not broken at all.

Be careful of thinking you are a certain way and that you will stay this way forever. Your life will change, your turn-ons will change. My friend Esther Perel brilliantly says, "We don't have one sexuality; we have multiple sexualities." I couldn't agree more. In my own life, my desires have shifted over the years. Allowing it to shift, allowing myself to integrate identities that have become fixed, and discovering what is unchangeable has been one of the most powerful steps in my sexual empowerment.

Some part of you is unchanging. That statement may seem to run counter to what I am saying above. But when you look inside, you'll find that you are both what changes and what doesn't change. Trust me, you'll soon understand what I mean, and in the long run, you'll have more sexual freedom— because you can play with any identity you desire!

Take a moment right now to reflect on these seven myths. What did you learn? Are you starting to have a different perspective?

Wonderful! Let's get you started on the next step of your sexy adventure . . .

Your Erotic Blueprint Breakthrough

One of the things I set out to do with the Core Erotic Blueprints was to create a new language for talking about love and sex. I wanted to give people a map to who they are so they could successfully communicate with one another about intimacy, arousal, connection, and sexual satisfaction.

Let's talk about pleasure.

Let's talk about our orgasms.

Let's talk about how we love.

The Erotic Blueprints give you a new language to share yourself and your turn-ons. They open the door to greater compassion for yourself and for others as we all navigate this sexual (r)evolution together. If we can talk together and seek to understand each other, that's a game changer.

So often we are looking for understanding, but we confuse that with compatibility or agreement. You and your partner(s) do not have to agree; you do not have to be "sexually compatible" in order to love each other and have a great sex life. But you do need to do your best to understand each other.

The biggest breakthrough I see people having when they learn their Core Erotic Blueprint is that they suddenly understand themselves. There's an aha moment of seeing that they are not broken, they are not incompatible, they don't deserve to be shamed because they don't fit the sexual norms.

The lightbulb of hope goes on.

This is a big step on the journey of sexual self-realization. You may have already had a few of those just by reading and doing the exercises in this chapter.

Are you starting to see the possibility that we aren't who we thought we were?

When we allow the fixed identity to fall away, something true emerges.

When you understand who you are and you *own* who you are, well . . . that's a total system reboot!

We can have compassion for each other because we now see that our partners aren't trying to hurt us or being stubborn, they just speak a different language than we do. They see the world through their filter, and we see the world through ours. It doesn't make anyone bad or wrong.

If we seek to understand their filter and to get to the bottom of what they truly need and desire, we can build our relationship on a new, authentic, and empowered foundation.

Journal Quickie:
Revealing Your Outcomes

Take a moment right now to write in your journal or share with a friend. What are the outcomes you wish to achieve by embarking on this journey? List at least ten outcomes you feel would make a difference in your sexual awakening.

Knowing your Core Erotic Blueprint gives you a map to your pleasure. And that map allows you to communicate your needs and desires to a partner whether you are newly dating or have been together since forever.

In the following chapters, I'll share the three pillars that shape your unique Core Erotic Blueprint map:

1. What is your Sexuality Stage or state?
2. What is your Erotic Blueprint Type? ·
3. What are the obstacles and pathways to your sexual health and wellness?

These pillars will give you a snapshot of who you are right now, at the start of your journey. You may find that by the middle of this journey, there are surprises; the terrain may not be exactly as you mapped it out to be. This pleasure map will lead you to deeper truths. There will be twists, and there will be things that take you off the map. You will find new friends and community, you will gain wisdom, and hopefully, you will truly meet yourself.

Let's get started with the first leg of your Core Erotic Blueprint journey: identifying your Sexuality Stage.

five stages of sexuality: which one are you living in?

We're now ready to begin creating your pleasure map . . .

There are five stages or states of sexuality.

I use the term "stage" to denote a longer amount of time you are in an experience of your sexuality, and "state" to denote a shorter amount of time. Think of it as being in a stage of life versus experiencing a temporary state or mood.

Do not think of these stages as hierarchical. They're all important, and each has its own Superpowers and Shadow side. But no one stage is better than the other, nor are we striving to get to the "top." You can find yourself fluctuating through all five states in a single day, or over the course of years. The key is to know where you are and if that stage is serving you and providing you with value, or if it's time to develop yourself in another stage.

Pleasure First: Stretch and Breath

The sensation of stretch can be highly pleasurable—let's see just how pleasurable it can be for you . . .

Begin by giving your body a big stretch, like when you first wake up in the morning. What can you do to make this stretch as long and luxurious as possible? Try stretching on your back first, then turn over and stretch on your belly. Maybe play with yoga poses, like Child's Pose or Mountain Pose.

As you stretch, ask yourself these questions: What would make this stretch even more pleasurable? What happens if you stretch one side of your body? What happens if you lie down or sit up or stand? Which position is most pleasurable for a stretch? How about just spreading your fingers or your toes or any specific part of the body you might enjoy lengthening? Begin to explore all your options.

Add breath by inhaling in through your nose as you stretch and then exhaling out of your mouth as you release the stretch. What happens when you add a big yawn to this stretch? What way of breathing makes your stretch most pleasurable?

What happens when you close your eyes and stretch? How about adding a sigh or a moan? What happens if you stretch and tense the muscles of your body while you hold your breath, then let everything go?

Keep exploring, listen to your body, and find what brings your body the most delicious pleasure right now, in this moment. Practice for at least fifteen minutes.

Notice how this practice makes you feel.

The five stages/states are:

» Resting

» Healing

» Curious

» Adventurous

» Transformational

Let's take a deeper look. As I'm describing them, think about which ones sound like where you currently are.

Take the following quiz and discover your Sexuality Stage, so that you know where you are on your sexual journey!

1. Which of the following describes your level of sexual knowledge?

   A. It's like a foreign language I once learned, but now I hardly speak it, or have forgotten how.

   B. I need information to help me move past what's blocking my sexual development.

   C. I want to know more, especially techniques to help me improve my sex life.

   D. I'm excited to explore "out of the box" concepts, so I feel like sex takes me to uncharted territories.

   E. I'm excited to learn how to use my sexuality for personal growth and development.

2. What is the quality of your current sex life?

   A. What sex life?

   B. In need of healing and with plenty of obstacles.

   C. Good, but I know there's more.

   D. Great! I'm having fun exploring.

   E. Spiritually enlightening—and I'm ready to soar even higher.

3. Pick a pair of words to describe your current sexual experiences:
   A. Distant or disconnected
   B. Painful or embarrassing
   C. Curious or fumbling
   D. Pleasurable or kinky
   E. Sacred or intimate

4. What is your number one sexual goal?
   A. To reconnect with my partner or to have a greater quantity of sex.
   B. To heal a past wound or to overcome a sexual issue.
   C. To learn how to improve my sexual skills and enjoy sex more.
   D. To explore all that's erotically possible or to learn something kinky.
   E. To experience the "more" to sex or to learn how to use sex as a tool for personal development or a connection to something greater than myself.

5. What best describes your comfort level with sexuality?
   A. Either my partner or I am not comfortable at all.
   B. I'm trying to overcome shame and guilt around sex, or sex is physically painful for me.
   C. I love asking questions about sex, or I read books and watch videos to learn more about sex.
   D. I can talk openly about sex with my friends and have no problem purchasing adult toys in a shop, or I am comfortable discussing taboo topics concerning sexuality.
   E. I am comfortable with sex as long as it is put in a sacred or spiritual context, or I am comfortable with Eastern ideas about sexual practice.

Tabulate your results by adding up the number of each letter you selected.

MOSTLY As—RESTING

You are in the Resting stage of your sexuality, which simply means you are not currently sexually active.

MOSTLY Bs—HEALING

You are in the Healing stage of your sexuality, and it's time for you to do what is needed to help your body, mind, or soul find healing.

MOSTLY Cs—CURIOUS

You are in the Curious stage of your sexuality, so it's time to learn as much as you can about sex and then put that into practice!

MOSTLY Ds—ADVENTUROUS

You are in the Adventurous stage of your sexuality, which means you are loving pushing the edges and exploring new things about your sexuality.

MOSTLY Es—TRANSFORMATIONAL

You are in the Transformational stage of your sexuality, which means you may be interested in what more there is to sex, and it's time to explore things like Tantra, Taoism, and other sacred sexual practices.

Now that you've taken the quiz, you can start to look closer at the five stages of sexuality to help you understand where you are and have more compassion for yourself. Remember that there is nothing wrong with any of these states, but knowing them is critical for mapping out your Core Erotic Blueprint.

Resting

The Resting stage is when you are not having sexual or erotic interactions. If you find your sexual activity is declining, you may be moving into the Resting stage. You may be resting if you find yourself in a sexless relationship. Or maybe you are simply resting because you feel content in your life and do not have any desire to have sex. Resting may also be the result of a conscious choice to practice celibacy. Perhaps, by choice, you've never had a sexual interaction in your life because you're waiting for the time that feels right for you.

There are times when we all need to rest, to be in stillness, and to rejuvenate ourselves. I often think of resting as an opportunity to hit the reset button on our sexuality. The problems occur when someone gets stuck there, especially if they're in a relationship with a person who is not in a resting phase of their own. Being in a sexless relationship with someone you love can cause a lot of distress. Resting is a natural part of our sexuality, but it can sometimes also indicate bigger health challenges, mental health issues, or problems within a relationship.

Resting often ties in with the next stage, healing, as sometimes we need to rest in order to heal. That can be a very positive thing for our bodies, minds, and souls. But if you've been resting for too long, it may be time to get back into the eroticism of life, either with yourself or with a partner.

Healing

In the Healing stage, you are likely recovering from something either physically traumatic or emotionally hurtful.

After the birth of my son, I was thrown into a Healing and Resting stage of my sexuality (the two stages often go hand in hand). I had suffered physical trauma. As I was giving birth, my pelvic floor was ripped through. It was nine weeks before I could think about having sex. My body needed to heal.

The Healing stage is a very important stage of our sexual lives, and you'll most likely experience a sexual healing event sometime in your life. Here are some examples of life events or physical factors that result in a Healing stage:

- » Fall or injury to your pelvis
- » Infection (UTI, bacterial infection, etc.)
- » Surgery (hysterectomy, etc.)
- » Childbirth
- » Menopause
- » STI/STD
- » Labial tears
- » Erectile dysfunction
- » Hormonal imbalance
- » Inflammation and pain
- » Vaginismus
- » Vulvodynia
- » Spinal injury
- » Adhesions and scar tissue

Keep in mind that this stage isn't just about your physical body but also your emotional well-being. You can be in the Healing stage if you are experiencing:

- » Deep grief
- » Heartbreak
- » Betrayal
- » Loss
- » Major life changes
- » New stress
- » Caring for a parent or sick loved one

» Recovery from sexual assault or acute trauma

» Anxiety

» Depression

» PTSD

» C-PTSD

If you are managing a condition related to your overall health or any kind of illness—physical, mental, or emotional—you are most likely in the Healing stage of your sexuality.

Just like with the Resting stage, there is value to allowing yourself the opportunity to heal. You do not want to rush your healing. This is an opportunity to listen to your body and to go slowly. This stage can be a great teacher, showing us what needs to change and transform in our lives. It can help us create healthier boundaries, teach us to ask for help when we need it, and allow us to develop a different kind of intimacy with ourselves and our lover(s). The problems arise when you don't want to take responsibility for your own healing, when you're unwilling to work with people who can care for and help you, or when you give up.

I've met clients who didn't want to get better or even work with their illness because they wanted to avoid having sex with their partners. They were stuck in the Resting stage, but were using the Healing stage to mask their lack of desire or even their feelings of disgust for their partner. Some people get stuck in the Healing stage out of concern for their partner's health. My client Cloe said she avoided sex with her husband because she had genital herpes. "I just don't want to risk giving it to him," she kept saying. She and her husband had been together for over twenty years; they had been sexless for almost five of those due to her recently more frequent outbreaks.

Cloe isn't alone; genital herpes infection is very common. The World Health Organization (WHO) estimated that worldwide, approximately 13 percent of people aged fifteen to forty-nine had HSV-2 (herpes simplex virus type 2) in 2022. The Centers for Disease Control (CDC) estimated that 12 percent of people aged fourteen to forty-nine had HSV-2 infection in the United States as of 2018.

Cloe's husband craved and desired her, and he made it very clear that he wasn't concerned about herpes. He loved her and wanted to be with her regardless of the virus. It wasn't just about intercourse for him. He wanted physical intimacy—kissing, hand holding, cuddling, skin-to-skin massages. Over the next four months, I would give them hundreds of erotic activities that they could play with. Many of these don't pose a risk of spreading the virus and didn't even have to involve Cloe's genitals.

It seemed things were good, and we were making progress—for a moment. "I just don't feel good now that I'm going through menopause," Cloe told me.

I felt compassion and care for her. And as we started to deepen the work, I noticed that she was resistant to trying anything that would create more physical intimacy between her and her husband.

"My back hurts too much" was the next one. Then the classic "I just get headaches every day, and I'm tired." Now my Spidey-Sense came online— something else was going on here.

One day, I simply told her, "Cloe, I'm starting to notice something that I'd like to share with you." She nodded.

"I'm noticing that every time we meet, there seems to be a new ailment or thing bothering you that you use as an excuse to not connect with your husband. What's going on?"

Then it all spilled out.

"I'm just not attracted to him anymore!" she said. "I don't want to have sex. I just want him to leave me alone!" A mix of tears and anger was rising as the truth came out. "I love him. I just don't want to have sex! It's so much easier to make it about my health than it is to tell him I'm not attracted to him anymore!"

And there it was. In almost thirty years of practice, I have never seen resistance be about the thing laying on the surface. Our resistance is usually centered around some truth we won't even admit to ourselves. If you're running around waiting until conditions are perfect to have an intimate life, you're most likely in some kind of resistance, and you've been lying to yourself about the truth.

Now, many people truly *are* in a healing phase—if you find yourself here and it's not resistance, it's time to get to work and help your body to heal. Rest may be the thing you need.

Just be sure that going deep into healing on your journey isn't really a way you're avoiding intimacy with someone you love. Many resources are available to you, as sexual wellness is rapidly becoming a more talked-about subject. Please be sure to check out the resources section at the end of this book (page 287) if you want more information on ways to begin your own healing process.

Curious

In the Curious stage of sexuality, you crave deep learning about how you can make sex even better. Curious can also have a contentedness to it, meaning that you feel well and good about your sex life and you're mentally, emotionally, and physically available to learn more. People in the Curious stage want to read all the books, take all the workshops, and learn as much "how to" as they can.

I speak at summits and workshops for many entrepreneurs and high performers, and I love asking them how many business books they've read. "Two hundred? One hundred? Fifty? Ten?" Most of the hands go up around the one hundred mark. "And how many workshops have you attended to improve your business or money skills? Ten, fifty, one hundred, over five hundred?" I love watching all the hands go up so eagerly and proudly. (The majority are in the hundreds.) Then I switch the topic. "Now tell me: How many of you have read a hundred books on sexuality?"

The audience is silent; no hands go up. "Fifty?" Still no hands. "Ten?" Now I start to get a few peppered throughout the room. "What books should we read?" someone shouts from the back row. So many of them are in the Curious stage for the very first time. I guarantee that within the next year, most of those people will have read at least a handful of books on sex or taken one of our courses or even hired a coach to show them the ropes—sometimes literally.

The beauty of this stage is that you can really dive into the wonderful world of learning everything you possibly can about sexuality. As you explore, you'll realize that sex is something you'll never stop learning about. When you gain skill sets around sex and learn how your own body loves to be pleasured, you increase your erotic intelligence, which leads to a much more fulfilling life overall! But the trap of the Curious stage is always staying in learning mode and never *applying* what you learn.

A book is safe, but it isn't real life.

Applying the practices and techniques in person that you've learned in theory requires courage and confidence. Take this book, for example. Have you actually done the Pleasure First exercises and all the exercises in the previous chapter? Or did you just read them?

Don't get stuck gobbling up content without putting it into practice!

Adventurous

The Adventurous stage of sexuality is one of expansion, play, getting out of your comfort zone, and exploring edges and new erotic possibilities.

Diane and Layla came to me wanting to have their first threesome.

They were terrified that it might mess up their amazing relationship, but they had both been fantasizing about it for years and felt it was time to go on a grand adventure.

"I really want to do this right," Diane said. "It feels like so much could go wrong. But we are so ready and turned on by the idea of bringing someone else into our bedroom! Can you help us do this, so it doesn't fuck up our relationship?"

How to have great threesomes, foursomes, etc., is a topic for another book, but if you're craving one, you just might be in the Adventurous stage! Adventure can stretch your sexual knowledge and skills, expand your ability to communicate, and allow you to play with more styles of Blueprintified Pleasure.

What grand sexual adventure would you love to go on? What have you yet to try from your sexual bucket list? Here are some adventurous ideas you might have considered:

» Getting new sex toys to try

» Having a threesome

» Attending a sex party

» Trying something kinky

» Playing out a fantasy

» Role-playing

» Having a one-night stand with a stranger

» Playing with a new sexual position

» Trying something you've always wanted to try but have been too scared to go through with

» Anal play

The challenge for many people in the Adventurous stage is that they tend to jump into their explorations without knowing how to play—and play safely—in this new way. You can end up making a lot of mistakes you'd rather avoid; for example, opening your relationship to additional partners without clear agreements in place beforehand, or diving into a new sexual experience with the wrong people. Most mistakes can be avoided with a little education. It might be time to step back into the Curious stage to learn how to expand and explore without doing harm to yourself or others.

One challenge of the Adventurous stage is that people often find themselves chasing more and more and more adventure. I see this in the entrepreneurs I work with; those in the Adventurous stage start to treat sex like an extreme sport: more ecstasy, *more* things they've never tried before, *MORE* peak experiences!

After big sexual expansions, it's good to take a break and integrate the experience and your new knowledge; otherwise, you just become an experience chaser. Remember, more isn't always better!

Transformational

When it comes to sex and pleasure, have you ever thought, *There's got to be more than this!* If you have, you just might be in the Transformational stage. This stage is all about what's possible with sex; it's the exploration of sexuality as a tool for spiritual growth, personal transformation, sex magic, and manifestation.

In the Transformational stage, you might find yourself:

» Curious about Tantric sex

» Interested in blending sexuality and spirituality together

» Studying what the Taoist masters had to say about sexual rejuvenation

» Diving into sexual magic and ancient practices from earth-based and Indigenous cultures

» Wanting to use sexuality to attain enlightened or ecstatic states of consciousness

» Experiencing meditation as equally, if not more, pleasurable than physical sex

If you find yourself interested in Tantra, Taoism, the practices of Quodoushka, the White Tigresses, or other ancient practices, you are in the Transformational stage. It's all about what else is possible and how we can use sexuality as a tool to realize who we are, experience mystical states of consciousness, and reach ecstatic heights of oneness and unity.

Sounds pretty good, right? Well, I'm a little biased. This stage is where I like to hang out a lot. As a teenager, while my friends were reading articles about the latest celebrity or how to do their makeup in teen magazines, I was researching ancient sexual practices from around the world and learning Tantric techniques to attain enlightenment through sex. I had a lot of the Curious stage, too, as I wanted to study everything I could about sexual practices and how they were linked to spirituality.

Perhaps it was my Catholic upbringing that had caused me to view sex as shameful and, eventually, to seek out a spiritual connection to sex. My thinking at the time was that if it was for a spiritual purpose, it couldn't be "bad."

The challenge is that you can end up chasing enlightenment, seeking and seeking and seeking and never having a direct experience of the enlightenment you crave. People in the Transformational stage can also gain a sense of superiority and think their approach to sex is superior, which is not the case. They can get judgmental of others and, thus, cause more separation instead of the unity these ancient practices were meant to create.

Now that you've taken the quiz and learned about each of the five stages, it's time to get honest with yourself about which stage or state you're in right now.

Journal Quickie: Exploring Stages

To dive deeper into your current stage of sexuality, answer the
following questions.

» *Which stage do you find yourself mostly in right now?*
» *How do you feel about being in that stage right now?*
» *Is there a stage you would prefer to be in, or are you
  content where you are?*

If there is a stage you would like to be in, write down a
few ways you could begin to explore that stage.

CHAPTER SIX

the five erotic blueprint types

I have a feeling you've had enough foreplay—now it's time for the main event. In this chapter, I'll share the basic essence of each Erotic Blueprint Type.

As of this writing, over two million people have been empowered by this sex-life-changing framework. They've discovered a new language that helps them articulate their needs and desires, their turn-ons and turn-offs—so they now live a sexually fulfilling life. They've discovered a new approach to sex and pleasure that allows them to own and enjoy who they are erotically. And they've gained confidence in their abilities to meet their lover's needs and fulfill their lover's deepest desires.

Would you like to experience this kind of transformation in your sex life? Get excited for the next big step on your erotic journey.

Pleasure First: Noticing
Your Pelvic Floor

The pelvic floor muscles surround your erectile network and support the vital organs. Having a healthy pelvic floor helps you have stronger orgasms and more pleasure in your genital area.

Tune into your pelvic floor and notice the sensations there. Do you feel the pressure of the seat beneath you or the texture of your clothing? Are you aware of sexual arousal or pulsating sensations?

There's no right or wrong thing to notice.

If you are a person with a penis, focus on the area between your scrotum and your anus. If you are a person with a vulva, focus high in the vagina near your cervix. Begin to squeeze and release this area of your body. Notice what arises with focused attention.

Ask yourself, *What would make this even more pleasurable?* Could you add some breath? Move slowly in circles or thrusts? Simply allow yourself to explore.

What would happen if you increased the speed of the contractions and relaxations while visualizing penetrating a partner or being penetrated? Does that increase or decrease pleasure? What would happen if you went even slower and more sensually? What would happen if you just imagined squeezing and releasing but didn't actually do it?

After several minutes of exploration, stop and notice your pelvic floor again. What has changed as a result of this practice?

You Are Not Broken

We talked about this in chapter four, and I want to keep reminding you: you—yes, *you*—are whole and complete.

As you read this book, doubts or fears might arise. Or you might have thoughts that it's really for someone else.

It's not. It's for you.

And if you haven't had those thoughts somewhere along this journey, you are one of the rare few who feels sexually confident, like anything is possible—and that's amazing! You know you aren't broken, you know that you can experience a whole world of erotic possibilities, and you know you are extraordinary and ordinary and "normal," all wrapped in one package.

And guess what? If you're reading this book because you think your lover is broken—they aren't broken, either! You can stop blaming them or thinking something must be wrong with them.

There isn't.

They might just be wired differently than you.

You've most likely heard the common refrain that we fear what we do not understand. Well, what I see around sexuality is that we judge what is different from what we know about our own selves. I invite you to stop judging your partner and start doing the work to understand them. Believe me, when you choose this path, it's a much more loving choice that creates a lot less suffering.

The five Erotic Blueprint Types help people understand that they are not broken or abnormal in any way. They give each of us permission to be our amazing erotic selves.

So far in this book, you've taken your first peek into who you are and what stage of sexuality you may be in. The Erotic Blueprint Types will help you see how you are erotically wired for your unique brand of turn-on, and that there is no shame in how you're wired. I think all the Erotic Blueprint

Types deal with shame about their sexuality, but remember: this work is all about knowing yourself and accepting yourself.

"I don't know, I just feel like I'm broken, and this is impossible. I'm never going to feel turned on or okay about my sexuality." This wasn't the first time Nellie had said these words to me. She was stuck in the belief that she was beyond repair in the sexual realm and that she had no interest in sex. And she felt shame about all of it. Part of Nellie's challenge was that she hadn't discovered what worked for her and what allowed her to feel good.

Of course she didn't want sex! Why would she, when nothing she had tried so far had turned her on?

"Are you willing to find out what turns you on, and to be surprised by it?" I asked her.

"Yes, but I'm a little afraid of being disappointed again. I mean, nothing— and I really mean that—nothing has worked," she replied.

At this point in a session, when a client and I are just starting to work together, it's important that I know what they've tried and what hasn't worked. I posed the question to Nellie.

"Well, I have mostly tried vibrators, intercourse, rubbing around naked, and I had a G-spot massage once," she replied, squirming a bit in her seat. "I've tried a few different sex toys, oral sex, and fingering. I've watched porn. It did nothing for me."

Right away, I could tell that most of Nellie's sexual explorations have been in one particular Erotic Blueprint Type. This is the case for many people: one Erotic Blueprint Type is being explored, leaving the other four completely out of the person's erotic expression. When they think of sex, they think of the standard narrative of sexuality, and they miss out on so much of what is there to play with, either partnered or on their own.

Nellie and I created a very safe container for her, so she could explore slowly and not repeat what hadn't worked for her in the past. I felt incredibly excited for Nellie, because I'd seen this so many times before in my practice. I knew that within the next three hours, Nellie would have an entire list of turn-ons because there was so much she hadn't explored. There are many, many layers to your sexual arousal, from who you are turned on by to what sensations turn you on and in which situations or contexts intimate encounters take place. I can assure you that none of this is the same for *everyone*.

Sure enough, after three hours of exploration with various touches in different Erotic Blueprints, Nellie sat there in tears of amazement. "I'm alive! I'm not sexually dead! How did I go so long not knowing this?"

I live for these moments of awakening.

"I'm so grateful right now to know that there are things that turn me on and that I can share this with someone," she said. She wiped a tear from the corner of her eye, which now had the unmistakable sparkle of someone who just met their erotic self.

I'm going to share how you can discover this for yourself and/or with a partner in chapter twelve, but first let's look at the Erotic Blueprint Types so you can begin to understand this revolutionary framework.

As you read this introduction to the five Erotic Blueprint Types, you may find yourself resonating with one or more of them. Most of us aren't strictly one type, but a combination of some or all five. Typically, though, you have a Primary Blueprint, where you find your easiest access to pleasure and turn-on.

As we explore the essence of each of the Blueprints, I'll often refer to its Superpowers and Shadows. Each type has its own Superpowers and Shadows, and you can have the Superpowers of one Blueprint and the Shadows of another. The Superpowers are where each type is wired to find pleasure with the most ease, the special forms of arousal and turn-on that light desire aflame; they define the pleasure sandbox in which each type most loves to play. The Shadows are elements that put the brakes on pleasure for each type. These can be emotional, physical, biochemical, or energetic (more on this later).

The Five Erotic Blueprint Types

THE ENERGETIC

The Energetic is turned on by space, teasing, anticipation, and yearning. They have some extraordinary Superpowers, like being able to have orgasms without even being touched. On the Shadow side, they can get caught in oversensitivity, which can create numbness and short-circuit their turn-on.

It just so happened that Nellie had a lot of Energetic in her Pleasure Profile. Most of her arousal came from *not* touching. That may sound confusing. How can you not touch and still create arousal, turn-on, and even orgasms?

You'll find out more about that in the next chapter.

THE SENSUAL

A Sensual is turned on by all their senses being ignited: a delicious taste, a favorite song playing in the background, the smells of sensuality, colors and flowers and setting—oh, and don't forget the style of touches: all over their body! Contouring touch. Melting, flesh to flesh!

A Sensual brings beauty to the erotic experience. Like Energetics, Sensuals possess the Superpower of being able to orgasm without genital touch. On the Shadow side, Sensuals are notorious for getting caught in their heads and not being able to relax into a sexual encounter.

We found out that Nellie had a hard time staying present during sex, which would plummet her connection to pleasure. Given the right context and exercises to help her find and meet sensation in her body, she was able to stay in the sensuality of the experience, surrendering and opening herself to pleasure.

THE SEXUAL

The Sexual is turned on by what most people typically think of as "sex." Give a Sexual nudity, genital touch, penetration, and orgasms, and all is right in their world.

A Sexual is most likely able to go from zero to sixty in no time. They are simple in their sexuality, but do not lack a feeling of depth.

The challenge with most Sexuals is that they miss the journey of a fully realized sexuality that invites and includes the pleasures of all the Erotic Blueprint Types.

Nellie was trying very hard to find turn-on in the Sexual Blueprint. She was trying what she thought should turn her on because she didn't know there were other forms of pleasure to try. It's an easy mistake to make. After all, we're told we should be turned on by genital touch and orgasms and sex toys and nudity—and for a Sexual, all these things work wonders! But most people need to explore other things before activities within the Sexual Blueprint will be a turn-on for them.

THE KINKY

The Kinky is turned on by taboo. And that can mean anything that is taboo for you: Love to be tied up or do lots of role-playing that feels naughty and edgy for you? You just might be a Kinky Type! If you've never had anything but missionary-style sex and getting a blow job feels taboo to you—you just might be a Kinky Type.

There are infinite ways to explore this Blueprint. Some people who are Kinky are more sensation-based (they love ropes and spanking, for example), while others are more psychological-based (they love role-play and power games, for example). And some Kinkys are both.

The Kinky's biggest Superpower is that they are endlessly creative and playful.

A common Shadow that Kinky Blueprints face is that they feel ashamed of their sexual desires because they're typically seen as taboo. In Nellie's exploration, she discovered that she was turned on by being objectified. This was very difficult for her to reconcile because she was a strong woman who didn't want to be objectified outside of the bedroom.

THE SHAPESHIFTER

The Shapeshifter is turned on by it all! They love it all, they want it all, and often they want a lot of it. They have a huge appetite and a broad palate for many forms of pleasure. If, as you were reading about the other four Blueprints, you found your desires represented in all the Types, you might be a Shapeshifter. This Blueprint is like all the other Blueprints rolled into one—plus some of its own unique characteristics.

The Shapeshifter is highly erotically intelligent. This often gets mistaken for being too complex or needy. The Shapeshifter can have many Superpowers, but one unique one is that they can shapeshift to please any lover—it's like being able to speak many languages fluently.

Nellie had the potential, as we all do, to become a Shapeshifter. However, she first needed to fully dive into the Blueprints in which she had easy access and connection to her own pleasure.

Trauma and the Erotic Blueprints

I define "trauma" as the way we adapt to adverse and intense situations. None of the Erotic Blueprints are immune to the effects of trauma, but after taking thousands of in-depth sexual histories, I have found that people who identify as Energetics and Sensuals tend to have the most unresolved trauma in their histories. And as a trauma-informed somatic sexologist, I find that many of them are still storing that trauma in their bodies.

Unresolved trauma or chronic stress can cause a person's nervous system to remain activated in a protective response, like the freeze, float, fawn, or flee response. In this state, a person sees most situations—even a partner who wants to be close—as a threat. This may cause them to avoid intimacy entirely because it doesn't feel safe. When someone's nervous system gets stuck in this response, they may be diagnosed with post-traumatic stress disorder (PTSD).

I believe that we live in a culture that creates trauma around sexuality. Very few people escape moving through this world without being shamed for their desires.

The #MeToo movement has shed light on how prevalent sexual abuse is in our culture. I set out on a mission years ago not only to help people who have been survivors of sexual abuse and trafficking, but also to prevent it. Putting an end to rape culture requires a collective change in consciousness, which happens only when we all take a stand together.

No more.

It's time.

It's well *past* time.

Breath is one way we can regulate our nervous systems and ground ourselves. So let's take a breath: Deep inhale. Exhale all the way out.

For some people, the mindfulness exercises in this book can be uncomfortable or cause anxiety. This may be due to a history of chronic stress, trauma, or other mental health challenges. Consider taking a titrated approach by doing a shorter version of the exercise or simply modifying it as needed (for example, keep your eyes open, or do the exercise in a location that feels safer to you than the location suggested). Over time, your body can build the capacity to experience pleasure!

Fight, Freeze, Fawn, Float, Flee, Fuck, or Feed

When the nervous system gets triggered, it can hijack us and cause us to move into certain responses. Notice if you have any of these responses when someone initiates sexual intimacy with you, or even during lovemaking.

FIGHT—Major bursts of adrenaline pour into your system, your heart rate increases, and you react by wanting to fight.

FREEZE—Your body freezes, tension comes in, and you react by playing dead.

FAWN—You do anything to appease the person you feel is a threat to you in that moment. You say yes when you really mean no.

FLOAT—This often accompanies a freeze response; you simply float out of your body and go numb so you don't feel what's happening.

FLEE—You run away as fast as you can. All the blood rushes to your arms and legs so you can get away from the danger and escape the scene.

FUCK—You get turned on when stressed or distressed and want to fuck aggressively to release that tension and find peace or relaxation.

FEED—When stressed, you react by turning to food for comfort and to calm your system; as a result, you overeat.

In chapter fourteen, we will revisit trauma and how it can put the brakes on your sexual wellness and pleasure. Please note that I am not a trauma therapist, and this book is not a replacement for therapy. If you've experienced sexual trauma in your history, please see the resources at the end of this book (page 287) for therapists who can support you on your journey.

This is just the beginning of your journey, so let's unpack each Erotic Blueprint Type in more depth and explore its Superpowers, its Shadows, and ways to really work with your own specific erotic wiring.

Prepare for your mind to be blown!

CHAPTER SEVEN

the energetic

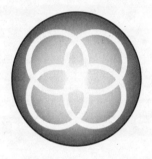

We are not just highly evolved animals with biological computers embedded in our skulls; we are also fields of consciousness without limits, transcending time, space, matter and linear causality.

—STANISLAV GROF

You Might Be an Energetic Blueprint If . . .

» Your turn-ons come from anticipation, space, and teasing. You love the foreplay more than the big event. You love the moment before the kiss.

» When physical contact is finally made and the space between is collapsed, you may be disappointed, and your arousal may flatline.

» You can feel unseen energies and are able to tap into spiritual dimensions; if channeled, these awarenesses allow you to experience cosmic and otherworldly orgasmic states.

» You consider sex a sacred act. You associate sex with spiritual pursuits and seek higher states of consciousness through your erotic practices.

» You can orgasm without even being touched. (Yes, it's possible.)

» You are highly empathic and often feel what other people are experiencing—both physically and emotionally.

» It may be difficult to say no to your partner, meaning you frequently put aside your own boundaries to avoid experiencing your partner's disappointment.

» You may consider yourself an introvert or a highly sensitive person. You are very sensitive to environmental stimulation, such as large groups and loud noises.

» If you are approached too fast or someone gets too close, too quickly, or you allow your boundaries to be crossed, you may mentally and emotionally check out or dissociate.

Imagine being teased until you are orgasming universes into existence with explosion after explosion of pleasure.

When it comes to experiencing all that is erotically possible, the Energetic Blueprint Type is one that will surely expand your ideas of sex, orgasm, and touch. And if you're reading this chapter and thinking that it sounds a bit woo-woo, that's okay. If you're feeling skeptical, I encourage you to suspend your disbelief for a moment.

If you think you must not be an Energetic because you aren't experiencing cosmic and otherworldly things, not to worry. There is a spectrum of development and growth for the Energetic Blueprint, and no matter where you are on that spectrum, you can expand into all that is erotically possible for you. You never know—you might be an Energetic and not even realize it!

If you already know you're an Energetic, I'm going to deep dive throughout this chapter into what is possible for you, and what your biggest blocks or Shadows may be to stepping into your full erotic potential.

And don't worry if you haven't figured it all out yet—we'll explore how to determine your Erotic Blueprint Type in chapter twelve.

The Energetic's Shadows

"Martina just isn't as into sex as I am. Every time I touch her, she freezes up or seems to float off somewhere."

I could feel Martina's whole body tense as her lover Kai wrapped his arms around her and squeezed her. She pulled away slightly as she tensed, and I could feel Kai's gesture was almost painful for her.

Her lover seemed oblivious to her response, even though his words told me he felt it and didn't know what to do.

Sadly, this is the challenge for a majority of Energetics. They have overridden their need for space so often that their bodies are stuck in a hyperalert state.

"I don't know what happens," Martina said. "I feel maybe a little turned on, but then it's like everything suddenly turns off and I just freeze. I go numb."

Maybe you can relate to this. You love the anticipation of sex, but when it gets physical, something in you just goes offline. Or maybe your body has gotten to the point where the thought of your partner initiating sex freezes you. Or, worse, any affection at all means there's pressure for you to have sex, so you've just stopped touching or desiring to be touched.

I'm sorry that you've never been honored for your unique form of arousal.

Don't worry, you are neither weird nor doomed.

As an Energetic, you have exquisite sensitivity, and once you cultivate your Superpowers, your orgasmic potential is vast.

A Shadow is something that creates distress or blocks a person from experiencing their full orgasmic and pleasure potential. Not all Energetics have Shadows, but it's important to be aware of them as you learn about this Blueprint Type. Here are some of the Shadows that are most challenging to the Energetic:

» Energetics may not set the boundaries and make the space that they need because they are trying to please a lover who wants more closeness. As a result, their body creates armoring and resistance to touch.

» Often they are haunted by some past trauma or intense experience that they haven't resolved.

» They can be so sensitive that too much, too fast will send them floating out of their bodies, and they will dissociate and lose all sensation and presence.

» They can get stuck in a hypervigilant nervous system response—flight, freeze, fawn, flee, or float.

» They are sometimes seen as cold, frigid, reserved, or not erotic.

» They can be incredibly judgmental of sexual interaction that they see as base, profane, or purely physical.

» They often feel shame because they are "weird" or outside of the box of what "normal" sex looks like in our culture.

Allow me to expand a bit on some of these Shadows.

Energetics Need to Just Say NO

Like Martina and Kai, couples will often blame each other for what isn't working. The Energetic blames their partner for always pushing sex, and their partner blames the Energetic for not being available for it.

The Energetic—in this case, Martina—constantly allowed her boundaries to be overridden and didn't know how to say no or state what she needed.

Her lover Kai missed the signs and assumed his partner didn't like touch or that something was wrong with her because she wasn't responding the way a "normal" sexual person should.

Blame exacerbates the disconnection. Blame creates more separation.

If you aren't necessarily turned on by touch, having a conversation about creating safety has probably been challenging. Energetics need a safe container.

They need space.

They need time to get into those ecstatic states.

But most Energetics do not know how to create that safe container, establish the boundaries they need to feel they can express themselves erotically, or pay attention to their body when it's saying "I need a pause" or even "I need to stop." They override themselves frequently.

Energetics have a hard time saying no because of their deep empathy. They feel what other people are feeling, and they don't want to hurt their partner. They don't want to ruin the moment. They don't want to seem "weird," so they just shut down and give over their body.

As a result, and over time, the Energetic's body armors itself more and more. They build up armor to affectionate touch. (Especially if their lover is a Sexual, the Energetic can be left feeling accosted over and over.) They become numb or dissociate in order to "get through" sex, which in turn creates more armor.

Often a deep root cause for Energetic Shadow is a past trauma or intense experience where it wasn't safe for them to say no. Perhaps in family dynamics, they were always overridden when they said no, or worse, they were abused for saying no. If there is sexual trauma in an Energetic's history, their "no" may have become a matter of life or death, and they had to dissociate to survive.

While an Energetic really needs to learn to say no and create healthy boundaries so that they can fully blossom into their highest states, many would also benefit from healing the past experiences that made their "no" unsafe to claim. Working with a therapist who specializes in trauma is highly recommended.

ARE ENERGETICS SEXUALLY FRIGID?

Energetics are often misunderstood by their lovers and viewed as cold, frigid, or just not "sexual."

This isn't true.

It's just the opposite.

They are so sensitive and so easy to turn on that they easily become overwhelmed by sensation and shut down. Arousal lives in the subtle realms for the Energetic. Some of the time, they are more turned on when there is a sense that they are out of their body.

Energetics can be highly erotic, just not in the way you might expect. The challenge of frigidity arises simply because no one has been taught how to play with an Energetic. No one has been taught that you can give someone a multidimensional third-eye orgasm that sends them off into the stratosphere.

Pleasure First: Energetic Eye Gaze

You can do this exercise with or without a partner.

Take a moment to close your eyes and simply follow the rising and falling of your breath.

Notice how pleasurable breathing is.

Can you stay with that experience for a moment?.

If you are practicing with a partner, open your eyes and make eye contact with them. Take a few breaths together.

If you're by yourself, sit in front of a mirror and make eye contact with yourself. Notice what happens as you make eye contact. Breathe.

Take your left hand and hover it over your heart or your partner's heart, keeping your hand from five to twelve inches away, without touching. If practicing with a partner, they can hover their hand over your heart.

Notice what feels good about this; notice if there is any anticipation of being touched.

Try this both with eye contact and with eyes closed, and notice which is more pleasurable for you.

After a minute or so of hovering touch, close your eyes again (if they were open). Return to your breath. Now scan for and notice pleasure in your body.

When you feel like you've completed the exercise, open your eyes. If you are single, thank yourself for doing this practice. If you're with a partner, thank them for this simple exchange of Pleasure First!

For Energetics who may have had a spiritual practice or energetic development, one of the Shadows I see most frequently (and one that I hate to admit I lived with for many years) is that they can get very judgmental about how they think sex should be. They may get rigid in their belief that sex always needs to be sacred or spiritual. They can get hierarchical thinking their way of being intimate is more spiritual than other people's, and that other people are base or profane. They may even believe that one should ascend past their physical body and their need for sexual connection.

I've even heard one client tell his partner, "I have sex in my crown chakra. You are coming from your lower chakras, and you are base and dirty." That was a surefire way to shame his lover and make her feel bad for her desires.

I really relate to this Shadow because after years of studying Tantric sex, I felt that sacred sex was the "enlightened" way. But judging or shaming others isn't so enlightened.

PLEASURE FOR PLEASURE'S SAKE

There are so many different expressions of sexuality, so many ways for us to experience pleasure in this life. I used to believe that pleasure for pleasure's sake was wrong. I felt safe having Tantric sex because it was spiritual, and therefore, it must be okay, but deep down, I was still harboring Catholic guilt. Once I realized this, I saw how judgment and shame showed up with my Energetic clients, too.

I'd been working with Jack and his wife, Shauna, for six months when he finally got it.

"Oh, pleasure for the sake of pleasure is okay!"

Before that moment, it was pleasure to become enlightened, pleasure to procreate, pleasure to be more of a man, pleasure to enhance their relationship. Once Jack finally realized this, he finally let go of the shame of just experiencing pleasure.

If you are harboring judgment, shaming your lover(s) for their "base" desires, or feel you are more enlightened than other people, then you may have some work to do.

Check yourself and make sure you aren't still hiding shame and judgment about your own sexuality and pleasure. Check yourself to make sure you aren't spiritually bypassing your own needs, wants, and desires.

You can unconditionally love others and feel one with them, and still have healthy boundaries. You have a human body—don't forget that. If you are constantly trying to ascend out of your body, you may want to look at why. Can you love your human self just as much as you love your divine self?

If you're an Energetic, you may have been judged in the past for being you. You may have been made to feel wrong for the reality you live in—a reality that includes energy fields, unity consciousness, strong boundaries around touch, orgasmic or ecstatic states, and other transpersonal experiences.

You may have been made to feel a little "crazy."

I'd like to propose that instead, you are extraordinary, and walking through this world as a very sensitive, empathetic person, you've just had to adapt to some adverse situations. You may want to get out of your body because in the past, it wasn't safe there. This is understandable.

It's time to love yourself right where you are.

The Energetic's Turn-Ons

There are infinite ways that an Energetic can experience turn-on. None of them are the traditional things you think of when it comes to arousal.

Here's a quick list of the Energetic's remarkable turn-ons:

» Spaciousness that allows the Energetic to anticipate, to yearn, and to long for your touch

» Subtlety; the brush of a fingertip, gazing into your eyes, the wind blowing across their skin
» Stillness and grounding
» Playing with polarities, or energies that feel like opposites
» Your attention and presence
» Feeling safe
» Being guided into expanded states of consciousness or mystical experiences

The Energetic Blueprint Type is turned on by having space, teasing, anticipation, and yearning. They love longing. They feel more pleasure with the super light, super slow touch of a fingertip on their skin. Or they may feel much more turn-on in keeping the space between themselves and their partner(s) rather than being directly touched.

An Energetic's pleasure can fully bloom only when it has all the space it needs.

If this is hard for you to imagine, take a moment to remember your first kiss with someone you really wanted to kiss. Remember the anticipation, the longing, the buildup, the feeling of fireworks in your body as your lips came near or you thought about kissing them.

The biggest turn-on for the Energetic is in that space—the space of anticipation—and feeling that energy.

I once had a client, Kat, who was most orgasmic when you were ten to twenty feet away, sending them energy or enticing them with your own sexy thoughts.

They would writhe and moan and go into so much ecstasy because of the distance. But if you got any closer, their turn-on would seemingly vanish. The sweet spot, the orgasmic spot, for Kat was if you stood many feet away. Literally *feet* away! Eventually, if their lovers stayed in the tease and antic- ipation, Kat would beg for them to come closer. Eventually, touch did feel delicious, but Kat needed time and space for that desire to unfold.

Embody It: Finding the Sweet Spot

This exercise is to help an Energetic determine how much physical distance they want or need. You will want a partner to help. This doesn't have to be a lover; it can be a friend you trust.

Stand at least five to ten feet away from each other. Look into each other's eyes and take a deep breath together.

The Energetic is in control, and gets to determine how close their partner is at all times. When ready to begin the exercise, the Energetic should say "yes." "Yes" means that their partner can take very slow steps forward until the Energetic says "no." When the Energetic says "no," their partner must stop walking toward them immediately. The partner will then thank the Energetic for making their boundary known. For the Energetic, hearing "thank you" helps validate their feelings and rewires their brain to feel comfortable with setting a physical boundary.

The Energetic must say "no" at least twice before their partner is close, in order to practice saying "no." The Energetic can also say "back up a step." They will keep saying "yes" and "no" until they find the sweet spot where their turn-on feels the best.

ENERGETICS LOVE THE STILL AND THE SUBTLE

If you really want to turn an Energetic on, use more artistic subtlety in your love-making. Energetics find pleasure in things most of us take for granted: a breath, a glance, the wind touching their skin, being teased but not touched, a deep gaze holding them while they move, having the space to go inside and get lost.

An analogy I love to use is that an Energetic is like a still pool of water reflecting the beautiful skies above. The turn-on is in feeling that stillness. After enjoying that stillness for a while, perhaps someone comes and barely dips their finger in the water so that the ripples spread out deliciously over the lake of their body. If you cannonball into the water, you'll overwhelm them and lose the subtlety and stillness.

We underestimate the power of stillness and subtlety to create arousal and excitement. I invite you to use these tools whether you are Energetic or not.

POLARITY PLAY: LIGHT AND DARK ENERGETICS

Energetics are turned on by playing consciously with polarities. During sex, are you aware who is the giver and who is the receiver? Who is in control of the play and who is surrendering themselves to it?

Over the course of my work with clients, I've realized that there are two different types of Energetics: light and dark.

Don't mistake light Energetic for good and dark Energetic for bad. There is no good or bad about these energies. They are just very different in their erotic approach.

With light energy, think love, light, joy, bliss, happiness, heart, sacred spaciousness.

With dark energy, think tease, anticipation, ravishing with your eyes, edgy intensity, stalking your prey.

My client Kat, whom you just met, was a light Energetic. They loved playing in the space where they felt safe, where there was loving energy all around them, where people were positive and soft. They loved crystals and the sounds of instruments like Tibetan singing bowls and chimes. They used words like "being in the heart space" to describe lovemaking.

My client Sophia was also an Energetic, but she loved dark atmospheric music, being teased to no end, and dark, moody environments. She liked tattoos and piercings and wore dark eye makeup. She was much more of a dark Energetic. Her energy said "Back off." If you gave her all that love and light, the crystals and the heart stuff, she would be very turned off. She loved to be the prey in erotic games, being stalked by her lover energetically (with consent, of course).

Light and dark can be fun to play with as opposite energies.

ENERGETICS LOVE YOUR PRESENCE

I always say that if I could teach people one thing to help them become better lovers, it would be presence.

Most people don't know how to be present with their partner(s) during sex, let alone how to stay so attuned that they know when to pause and when to slow down.

Energetics crave their lover's full presence. They want their lover present with them in full awareness of this moment, here and now. Learning to be fully present with your Energetic lover will benefit your pleasure as well. It's one of the great gifts that the Energetic can give you.

And here's a tip: Keeping all your sexual hunger fully turned on but not acted upon is especially hot for Energetics.

This is quite the skill.

Can you turn your turn-on all the way up but resist taking any action to relieve it? When your hunger for your Energetic lover is apparent but you let them come to you when *they* are ready, it will rock their world!

SAFETY IS SEXY

If you are Energetic, ask yourself, *What could help me feel safer during sexual play?*

What do you need to communicate to a lover to help them help *you* feel safe? What kind of container would you like created for you so that you can go into your full erotic expression?

Energetics will fly super high the safer they feel. Grounding and presence bring safety.

What is grounding? Grounding can be as simple as holding the feet or the hip bones, or even resting the full weight of your body on someone. You can also use weighted blankets. This may seem counter to the idea of giving an Energetic space, but once they are flying off into the cosmos, touch that is still, present, and held with the intention of grounding can help an Energetic feel safer to reach the heights of ecstasy and deeper enjoyment. And it's not that Energetics don't like touch—they love it, especially if it's subtle, light, slow, energetic, and filled with teasing.

TO INFINITY AND BEYOND

For seasoned Energetics, expanded states and uncovering all that is erotically possible are huge turn-ons. An Energetic finds it easy to access ecstatic, unordinary, or transpersonal states of consciousness. They can achieve these states through pleasure, sex, and orgasm (and a variety of other tools, such as breathwork and meditation). The more you develop as an Energetic, the more likely you are to experience these ecstatic states.

Sexuality and eroticism are integrated with spirituality as a path of transcendence and growth in Eastern spiritual practices such as Tantra, Vajrayana, Buddhism, Taoism, and Kundalini yoga. These revered traditions unite sexuality with body, mind, and spirit. Western religious and spiritual traditions, on the other hand, have attempted to separate spirituality from the physical experience of sex, causing shame and disconnection within us.

The study of transcendent sexual and erotic experiences is growing. It seeks to investigate how a regular practice may open and allow someone to develop more expansive sexual experiences. I truly hope we see more research on this in the years to come. Until then, my personal experiences and those of my clients will have to suffice.

I was with a lover of mine named Michael Ashley.

He knows how to take me way out into expanded states during our erotic play, and we have traveled there together many times.

I was feeling, at the time, like I was on the verge of an explosion in my body, on the edge of birthing something new into the world. Have you ever felt the anticipation of launching a creative project out into the world? It was like that, only a hundred times more intense.

Michael Ashley began to stroke his fingertips energetically over my skin. So slowly, paying such deep attention to every quiver. Before I knew it, I was spilling into energetic orgasms, where I stayed for a long moment before he picked me up and put me on the bed.

I started to breathe up the front channel of my spine into the top of my head and then to make a vowel sound down the back channel of my body and into his mouth. He sucked at my sound as I released the vibration from my throat and opened my sex.

I started to have a cathartic orgasm. Laughing and crying. My body writhing in so much ecstasy. But there was still so much pent-up energy.

Somehow, he knew what to do. He pressed his forehead right into my pelvic floor, and it was like the floodgates opened. It was like I was giving birth to an entire universe right into his third eye.

He held me there as I poured into him with a release unlike anything I'd known. Weeping as I gave birth to this orgasmic universe. Laughing at the ecstasy of such a huge release.

It just kept coming and coming.

I started to breathe again, up the front of my spine, over my crown, and then down the back channel of my spine into him. Over and over until I was empty.

So empty—what a glorious release!

"Hold me," I said. He came up to the bed and wrapped his body tight around me.

Embody It: Gaining Awareness

This exercise is for lovers of Energetics to gain deeper awareness. You can do this exercise with a partner or with your own body! It will help you to increase your ability to hold presence, both with yourself and with another person.

Set a timer for fifteen minutes. During this period, you will explore a specific part of your body—your forearm, for example. If you have a partner, choose an area on their body.

Give that part of the body full presence.

This practice is all about noticing when your mind starts to wander and you lose full present-time awareness.

Look at their forearm (or your own) and notice the texture of the skin, the hairs on the arm, the skin tone. Look at it as if you were looking at a work of fine art you've never seen before.

Fifteen minutes can feel like a long time for some people, so you may want to touch lightly with your fingertips (remember, you are dipping into a still pool of water, so go light, go slow, and practice stillness).

Notice your breath.

Notice what sensations, thoughts, or emotions arise as you hold this presence with yourself or your partner.

After the timer goes off, journal about your experience, or if you're with a partner, take time to share what this experience was like for you.

Each time you do this, you will notice more and more subtleties and gain increased presence.

"I have a story," I told him. "Remember when we were stars deep in the universe, and we decided to become human so that we could do *that*?!" I laughed and laughed.

He just held me tighter.

I wept.

"This is why I never did psychedelics when I was younger—I had this!" I said. I laughed again, remembering experiences like this that I'd had in my teens and early twenties.

He laughed with me this time, his body absorbing more energy and waving in time with mine.

The night went on like this, wave after wave after delicious wave of Energetic play. All time lost. All space expanded.

I'm continually amazed at what is erotically possible.

Never stop exploring.

That was a new one—the *"birth a universe into your lover's third eye and remember you are a star" orgasm*!

What?

If you are an Energetic, you may understand what I'm referring to here; otherwise, my experience with Michael Ashley may be difficult to relate to. This type of erotic interaction, however, is not unique to us. I've worked with many people who have had transcendent sexual experiences without fully understanding what was happening.

I always feel a little vulnerable sharing my own big orgasmic Energetic expansion stories—this feeling is common for an Energetic, as sharing means they run the risk of being misunderstood. Once I spoke in an interview about how when we share what we have experienced during sex and intimacy, we open new possibilities for other people—for everyone—to have that experience. Even though I have niggling thoughts about how weird it all sounds to some people, or how it may be perceived in a less positive light, I feel that sharing this with you opens a door.

But don't take my word for it—the work of Stanislav Grof, a brilliant psychiatrist and pioneer in transpersonal psychology, may explain a lot of what Energetics experience. In his groundbreaking research, Grof found that many people have access to these multidimensional realms and to the states of consciousness that take them there. Grof is most known for his research into the use of expanded states of consciousness for the purposes of exploring, healing, growth, and insight into multiple dimensions. He coined the term "holotropic," which means "moving toward wholeness." His work with states of consciousness, psychedelics, and holotropic breathwork seeks to enable people to embrace their wholeness. He shares his personal experiences in many of his books.

"My consciousness expanded at an inconceivable speed and reached cosmic dimensions," Grof writes in *The Way of the Psychonaut: Encyclopedia for Inner Journeys.* "I lost connection with my everyday identity. There were no more boundaries or differences between me and the universe. I felt that my old personality was extinguished and that I ceased to exist. And I felt that by becoming nothing, I became everything."

Certain sexual experiences, similar to holotropic breathwork, also provide a way into these mystical states that Energetics seem more able to access. I personally have had the same exact experience that Grof describes having himself in his book.

The Energetic's Superpowers

There I was, blindfolded, writhing in orgasm in front of a thousand people, while Ian played my body without touching it. This is one of our most loved demonstrations: the Touchless Energetic Orgasm! We demonstrate this because once someone sees what is possible, it suddenly becomes real in their minds.

I don't demonstrate to show off, or so people feel they need to strive for something if they aren't having this kind of orgasm. No, I do it to show people what's possible when those who are the Energetic Blueprint Type fully cultivate their orgasmic Superpowers!

When I was first starting my career, I had a mentor named Kenneth Ray Stubbs, who wrote the book on erotic massage and has numerous courses on sexual shamanism and Tantra. Kenneth, who is paralyzed, wanted to explore what it would be like to have orgasms in various energy bodies without touch. We would sit across from each other and use visualizations to inspire pleasure and movements of orgasmic energies. This experiment taught me so much about what is possible.

We could just use an intention to create orgasm.

We didn't even need to be in proximity to each other. We could do this from anywhere, at any time.

This was my first dip into my own Superpowers as an Energetic and helped me fully develop into who I was as an erotic being. There was a part of me that wanted to prove that what I was experiencing was "real," so I turned to science to see if there was any proof of the existence of energetic fields.

I'm not a scientist, but for anyone who doubts what I'm suggesting, just know that there are ways to measure the bioelectromagnetic fields around the body. Bear with me as I get a little geeky here (maybe some of you are like me and are turned on by big science-y words—you might be an Energetic if the sound of certain words turns you on!).

Biomagnetics is the study of magnetic fields produced by living organisms. Biomagnetic fields are caused by electrical currents in conducting body tissues such as the heart or brain. In short, the human body produces electrical fields, and those fields are measurable.

To study these fields, scientists have created powerful measuring devices with something called a SQUID (short for superconducting quantum interference device—now *that* really turns me on). One measuring technique that uses SQUID technology is called (oh, you are going to *love* this word) magnetoencephalography, or MEG for short, and is a neuroimaging system that can detect biomagnetic fields in the brain. In essence, these devices prove that energy fields exist and that they are measurable.

I believe that Energetics are more attuned to these fields, both in their own bodies and in the bodies of other people. They can feel them and experience them more fully than people who aren't Energetic. When an Energetic is fully developed and owns who they are, their sensitivity to these fields gets even stronger.

And let's not forget that when we look at energy medicine, there are whole areas of study and wellness that have mapped out Energetic anatomy. Modalities including Ayurveda, acupuncture, acupressure, and pranic healing can teach us about these fields and the effects that touch, diet, and stress have on them.

If you or someone you love is Energetic, I highly recommend that you learn about energy meridians in both Chinese medicine and yogic practices from India.

Now that I've fed a part of your science mind, let's immerse ourselves in some of the fabulous Superpowers of the Energetic.

Here's a quick list of Energetic Superpowers:

» You can have touchless or energetic orgasms. Yes, it's true!
» You are very attuned to your lovers and can be present to everything you are feeling.
» You are hypersensitive—if done right, it doesn't take much to get you writhing in orgasmic ecstasy.
» Sex can feel like an out-of-body experience.

» You may experience synesthesia and taste music or hear color, which can also lead to orgasmic experiences.

» You can access holotropic or expanded states of awareness.

The Superpowers of the Energetic are remarkable. Especially when it comes to holotropic or expanded states of awareness. This phenomenon can seem strange to your lovers if they haven't experienced those states themselves.

If you are an Energetic who moves into expanded states, you may also experience a big emotional release during sex—do not get freaked out. Allow the emotions to flow. Say yes to the big energies moving through you. These are cathartic orgasms.

Many phenomena can come with big emotional cathartic orgasms. These experiences might look like your eyes rolling toward the back of your head. You might have spontaneous uncontrollable body movements (note to lovers: Energetics may not even be aware they're doing it), shaking all over your body, tingling in your hands, or undulating waves through your spine.

You might see visions, experience other lifetimes, have enhanced perception, speak in strange languages, travel beyond space and time, have complete mystical experiences (oneness, timelessness, the ineffable, etc.). You may repeat the same phrase over and over, sing, cry, experience memories you'd locked away—the list goes on.

If you are Energetic, you may be so empathetic and attuned that sometimes you can't tell if the physical sensations and emotions you experience are yours or your lover's. This can be fun when a lover is having an orgasm and the Energetic starts to have one, too. This can be difficult if the lover is distressed or distracted.

If you haven't unlocked these Superpowers yet, just remember that there is nothing wrong with you. You are whole and complete just the way you are, and if you want to put cherries, chocolate, and maybe some cosmic sprinkles on top of your erotic ice cream sundae, I'm here to show you how.

So Your Lover Is an Energetic . . .

If you have an Energetic lover, there are a couple of things that can make all the difference in deepening your connection.

First, create safe spaces for them, where they can be themselves and play all the way to the realms of erotic possibility. If your Energetic lover reports to you that they had one of these powerful transpersonal experiences, be supportive and stay open-minded. Listen to what your lover has to say. If you can't relate to or understand what they've experienced, do not make them feel wrong or "crazy" about what happened. These phenomena are quite extraordinary, and can be very meaningful for Energetics. It's vital that you validate their experience.

Second, really take the time to learn about energy, even if you don't believe in it yourself; take a class, start practicing energetic touch, or study books about transpersonal psychology.

These two things will go a long way to feeding your Energetic partner.

Where to Begin If You Are an Energetic

If you feel you may be an Energetic, I have three guidelines for you to begin with.

1. CLEAR YOUR SHAME.

If you want to grow into your full potential as an Energetic, the first step is to clear any shame about who you are and then to say "YES!!!" to the adventures that await you—no matter how out of the ordinary they seem.

Embody It:
Increase Your Capacity for Pleasure

If you begin to feel overwhelmed, here are more ways you can assimilate and increase your capacity for more pleasure. Practice this with a partner or on your own.

» **SPACE**—Get physical space, stop touch, and go to your sweet spot. Once you feel like your overwhelm has subsided, you can return to touch and sexual play.

» **SPREAD**—Use your hands, breath, movement, or visualization to move the sensation all over your body. Keep doing this until the overwhelming energy dissipates.

» **STILLNESS**—Stop what you're doing and just hold in stillness until your body feels ready for more. This can be done with still and grounding touch, too.

» **SOUND**—Make sound, such as big moaning, roaring, or humming noises, to help move and dissipate the overwhelming sensations.

» **SILLINESS**—Laughter can be a great way to transmute the intensity.

With practice, utilizing space, spread, stillness, sound, and silliness (or any combination of these) will help you meet overwhelming or intense sensations and be able to receive more and more pleasure.

You are amazing! You are incredible! You have a glorious sexuality that can take you to realms unknown to many. Do not be ashamed of who you are.

However, right now, you may not believe all this is possible for you and that's okay.

2. CREATE SAFE BOUNDARIES.

It's okay for you to say no.

And if you're in a relationship where it isn't safe for you to say no—it might be time to reevaluate that relationship. If you are truly unsafe, it's time to get out and get help immediately.

Before you play erotically, tell your lover(s) what you want to explore and share your boundaries with them. It's always acceptable to say that you don't want penetration, or even touch. Establish with your partner that you will inform them if it's too much or too fast. Create a safe container and be clear when making your needs known.

3. LEARN HOW TO ASSIMILATE SENSATION.

You are very sensitive, and sometimes that can be overwhelming. If you go into an unusual state of consciousness and you've never been there before, it can even be frightening.

Not to worry—you can learn how to assimilate or digest more and more sensation so that your system doesn't go into overwhelm and short-circuit.

Deep breaths can be a huge help. Looking into your lover's eyes as they hold you in stillness can be very powerful.

Now you've had an introduction to one of the Erotic Blueprint Types, I know you must be hungry for more.

If you're an Energetic, you could tease yourself by putting the book down for a day, but leaving it somewhere you can see it. Begin to wonder what is next. Count down the time until you get to read more. Imagine what pleasures may await you on the pages that follow . . .

Sensuals, mmmmmmm—you're up next.

Grab something tasty, maybe pour yourself a glass of wine or put on a delicious scent, and get cozy, because we're going to dive into all the delights that make you so scintillating.

CHAPTER EIGHT

the sensual

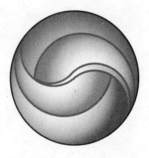

I want to be the first thing you touch in the morning
and the last thing you taste at night.

—SADE ANDRIA ZABALA

You Might Be a Sensual Blueprint If . . .

» You bring artistry to your intimate encounters.

» Sights, sounds, textures, tastes, smells, and touches can inspire turn-on and ignite your desire.

» You experience orgasmic sensations when tasting a delicious food, listening to an exhilarating song, smelling intoxicating aromas, rubbing rich textures on your skin, or surrendering into a lover's penetrating and connected touch.

» You can experience full-body, nongenital orgasms.

» You need to relax before your body and mind can open to arousal and erotic connection. You need transition time between your busy, stressful day and intimacy with a partner: a moment to make sure your checklist is done for the day, a warm bath, a nap, or time to cuddle.

» Sometimes cuddles, hugs, and kisses are enough to have you feeling fulfilled, and intercourse isn't even needed for you to be sexually satisfied.

» Your orgasm is sometimes elusive, or it may take longer than you expect to reach orgasm or ejaculation.

» You lose connection to your pleasure because your monkey mind distracts you: *There are socks on the floor. I forgot to make that phone call. How do I smell down there? I'm taking too long. How does my butt look in this light?*

» Any little distraction can seem to flatline your arousal.

Take a breath and notice any smells that bring you joy. Touch a curve on your body. Run your tongue around your mouth and notice any tastes there. Look around and find two or three things that please your eyes.

Welcome to the delicious world of the Sensual!

Sensuals love having all their senses ignited, and they love beauty in all their erotic encounters. In this chapter, I'll be sharing ways to slowly unfold the Sensual's turn-ons, and explain how Shadows block them from the profound Superpowers that leave them in full-body ecstasy.

Are you cozy? Does your environment feel delicious right now?

If so, let's go!

The Sensual's Shadows

"I don't understand what's wrong with me," Jackson said with a pained look on his face. "I mean, my wife is so hot. I find her attractive and I want to have sex with her. But something in my head won't let go."

"Go on, say more. Can you give me an example?" I asked him.

"Well, the other night, she was lying there naked on the bed. Look at her, she's gorgeous! And all I could think about were the socks on the floor. And the socks on the floor made me think about the laundry that needed to be done. And the laundry that needed to be done made me think about the kids, and all the millions of things I needed to do. And that led to making sure that I'm providing for our household and am I working enough? . . . Blah, blah, blah, blah, blah. See my problem? So instead of having sex with my beautiful wife, I'm all in my head, thinking about a million and one things that are not a turn-on!" Jackson was barely breathing when he was done, and his face looked tortured.

Maybe you can relate to Jackson.

Pleasure First: Connecting with Your Sensational Senses

Look around the space you are in and ask yourself how you can incorporate more sensuality into your surroundings. Start with simple things like picking up clutter, lighting a scented candle, making your bed, or bringing in some fresh flowers.

Take five to fifteen minutes to create a play space for pleasure, because for a Sensual, setting is everything!

Now put on a song that you find very sensual. You may even want to create a playlist of three to five songs that make you slow down.

As the song comes on, close your eyes and take a deep breath. Start moving. This might be simply swaying and feeling your feet on the floor or rolling your neck or moving your hips to the music. Now add touch to this experience. Let the music guide your hands over your body. Maybe you want to lie down or sit as you touch your skin, gliding your hands over every curve and crevice.

Keep breathing, stay focused on the music, and keep touching your body. You can include your genitals in this exercise, but don't focus all your attention there. Notice what brings you the most pleasure. Take a whole song to touch and move and breathe.

"That sounds really hard. Can I share some simple solutions with you?" I asked.

His face brightened.

Hope!

You're about to get intimate, and instead of being able to focus on the pleasure before you, it's like everything in the room starts talking to you—the crooked pillow, the unmade bed, the clutter on the nightstand, the clothing on the floor, the lighting that isn't quite right, the stack of things to do.

Or maybe it isn't so much about the things in the environment—maybe it's that you just don't feel in the mood because you have a hundred and one things on your mind and even more on your to-do list.

There you are, doing the dishes or folding the laundry or getting the kids to sleep, when your lover comes up behind you and whispers something sexy.

Instead of melting into them, tension rises in you, and you think, *Sex? Great, another thing to add to my to-do list before I can get to sleep.* You just don't feel relaxed enough to have sex in that moment, or in most moments, if you're being honest with yourself.

Sometimes this endless chatter in your head comes in the throes of passion. There you are, with your lover between your legs, and the tape starts to play.

Is everything okay down there?

I hope I smell/taste/look okay.

Oh no! I forgot to call [X] today. I need to remember to do that.

It's been a while and I still haven't had an orgasm. I'm taking way too long! Maybe I should just fake it and get this over with already!

What's today? Oh yeah, Tuesday. I need to make sure I have cheese sandwiches packed for lunch tomorrow. Wait, why am I thinking of that right now?

I think I need to pee/fart/burp. Oh God, I hope I don't pee/fart/burp!

This mind chatter can go on and on and on and on. It's what keeps you from being present with yourself and with your lover. It interferes with your ability to submit to pleasure in your body.

As a Sensual Type, getting caught in your head is the number one way to turn yourself off. When you don't tell your lover you're feeling this way, it can be a way to avoid intimacy and connection.

I'd say that for most Sensuals, this is the most common Shadow element that they deal with. Their brains just won't turn off.

Here are some other main Shadow aspects of the Sensual Type:

» The Sensual can get grossed out by mess, especially when it comes to bodily fluids.

» Unless everything is "just right," they can't let go and relax into the sexual experience.

» They "yuck" someone else's turn-ons and get judgmental about bodies, smells, and the way things look, and they can be cruel when they encounter these triggers.

» They need relaxation, comfort, and safety, and they often expect the external world to meet those needs instead of learning how to generate those feeling from within.

» They often act as a caretaker for everyone else and forget to care for themselves.

» Orgasms for Sensuals can seem elusive, like you almost get there but then the orgasm fades away. Sex can become a chase for pleasure instead of a luxurious enjoyment.

Remember Jackson? He was really grappling with Sensual Shadows. They came spilling out of him in our intake session. Now that the truth was out, it was like Jackson couldn't give me the whole story fast enough.

"And that's not all! When Makayla is going down on me, I can't focus at all. It's like I just can't accept that she'd enjoy that. I just think about how uncomfortable it must be for her, and I feel like I need to take a shower in case I'm sweaty and smelly. It's no wonder I can't get hard!"

The tension in the room was thick . . .

I could see the hurt in Makayla's eyes. Jackson tensed his jaw and his hands. This was a big pain point between them.

"He's fine," Makayla said. "I don't know why he's so worried about everything. I don't care. I just want to have sex with my husband. I don't get why I'm not attractive enough or skilled enough to get his mind off things." Her eyes began to well up with tears, and I could see Jackson beginning to move into a caretaker role.

"It's not your fault, baby, I swear. It's me." He pulled a tissue from the box and handed it to her, his focus shifting from himself to her.

It's very common for someone who loves a person stuck in a Sensual Shadow to feel hopeless, like they can't do anything right. They commonly feel like they will never be attractive enough or good enough for their partner. It can be so frustrating.

I know this pain firsthand.

My lover Ian struggled with Sensual Shadow a lot when we first met.

He didn't like mess, and I was an ejaculator who loved being in the soup of what I called "pleasure wetness."

I was ready to go 24-7. He needed to relax to have sex.

I was impatient and couldn't understand why he wouldn't just let it all go to be with me in the moment. He had a hard time transitioning from work into sexual play.

I was all good for quickies at any time. He wanted time to luxuriate together and to follow whatever feelings and impulses arose.

My libido ran high, and I wanted sex two to three times a day. His libido was lower, and sometimes snuggling together was all he needed to feel connected and satisfied.

He often took care of me instead of taking care of himself. He became a caretaker instead of a lover, which led him to desire less sex with me.

This all left me feeling unattractive, undesirable, frustrated, and, I hate to admit, angry. It was so hard for me to understand.

In my mind, all he needed to do was to let go of what was happening in his own mind. He needed to de-stress and get present. But that was so much easier said than done.

At times I lost my ability to have empathy for where he was. And I had to find understanding again and discover what I could do to help him, even if it took forty-five minutes of straightening up the bedroom and getting a multitude of little things done for us to get there.

I really had to learn to be patient and to help him create a sensual space for us to be able to come together.

Your Friend the Vagus Nerve

Vigilance is your body's natural way of adapting to stress to survive. Hypervigilance is an elevated state where we perceive that there may be some kind of danger or potential threat around us, even when there isn't. In this state, our nervous system is on high alert and does not have the capacity for pleasure.

We all experience stressors. As a world culture, we have gone through pandemics, wars, economic hardships, and environmental disasters, and these stressors and traumatic experiences create hypervigilance in our bodies. If we do not know how to calm ourselves or how to get out of the hypervigilant state, it can start to stick, and eventually becomes our normal state. Our bodies don't know how to relax anymore.

If you are stuck in this place, it can be hard to let your defenses down. You may find yourself feeling exhausted because your body is running off cortisol and stress is what feels normal. Yikes!

The last thing you think of is sex and intimacy. You may be in a state of fear, worry, anxiety, even paranoia. Your breathing may get shallow, your heart may race, you might break out into a sweat.

Embody It: Christian's Vagus Nerve Hum

Make yourself comfortable in either a seated position or lying with your back flat on the floor.

Bring awareness to your breath—without feeling the need to adjust, fix, or manipulate it, or to be a "good breather." Watch yourself breathing for three to five breaths.

Purposefully engage your breath slightly more deeply by imagining that your breath could fill your lower back. Expand into the back of your chair or down into the floor.

Allow your lips to gently connect with one another and begin collecting vibration to create a gentle hum. Think of the old Campbell's soup commercials: "M'm! M'm! Good!"

Sustain the hum on a single pitch several times. Change to a lower pitch and sustain it there several times. Change to a higher pitch and sustain it there several times.

As much as possible, let yourself focus on the sensation of the vibration rather than the sound being produced. If the hum feels tight, take a breath, change the pitch, or do less.

If you aren't feeling vibration on the lips, check that your tongue is soft and flat in your mouth and you aren't closing off your mouth with the back of your tongue, making an *ng* sound, or the tip of your tongue, making an *nn* sound.

Play subtly with the distance between your molars to discover the space that creates the most vibrational sensation on your lips. As you take a few gentle breaths, notice how your face and body feel different from when you began this Embody It practice.

It didn't surprise me to learn that my client Jackson was a veteran. He had served in Iraq. He had been diagnosed with PTSD and was in treatment to help him calm his nervous system, which was on overdrive.

When he came home from the service, he didn't know how to let down the part of his nervous system that had adapted—and rightfully so—to the high-danger situation he had been in. His PTSD was contributing to the Shadow side of his Sensual Blueprint, so I introduced him to something called polyvagal theory. We worked together with his team of coaches and therapists to help him learn to regulate his system.

The vagus nerve (also known as cranial nerve X) is the longest cranial nerve that we have and is the main nerve of the parasympathetic nervous system, which is responsible for the digest-and-rest part of our system. When you "tone" your vagus nerve, it's like working out a muscle. With increased tone, your body can relax faster after stress,

Dr. Stephen Porges, who developed polyvagal theory, conducted detailed research into the social functions of the vagus nerve. He found interactions with other people can increase vagal tone and calm the activated part of the nervous system.

Since the vagus nerve connects to so many parts of the body, it is possible to activate it indirectly through these points in the body. That means there are several things that naturally stimulate the vagus nerve and increase its tone. Some of these include exposure to cold, slow diaphragmatic breathing, meditation, vocalization (singing, humming, gargling, and laughing), and, exciting for us, sexual intercourse.

Singing can activate the vagus nerve via the muscles in the back of the throat and the inner ear. It's one of my favorite ways to stimulate this nerve, which is why I work weekly with Christian Duhamel, a voice and expression expert and Certified Erotic Blueprint Coach, to train my nervous system to stay calm. Plus, I love to sing.

"Singing is one of our birthrights as humans," Christian explained to me during a lesson. He told me about a study by Lucia Benetti which demonstrated that some babies even sing before they speak, repeating simple melodies, the lyrics to which they can't yet understand or pronounce. The vagus nerve innervates a number of critical organs in the body, including the muscles of the larynx (voice box). "By gently humming or lightly singing, each of us can use our body's natural abilities to move from sympathetic nervous system activity to the parasympathetic resting state. So if you ever feel yourself being activated by the circumstances around you, you can counteract that experience by bringing attention to the breath and engaging the voice with some gentle humming," says Christian.

The Sensual's Turn-Ons

Sensuals are turned on by having all their senses ignited. They are turned on by smells, sights, tastes, sounds, touches; all of these, if delivered just right, add to their erotic delight.

If the Sensual is tense or uptight, sex is the furthest thing from their mind and body. Sensuals need to relax for their body to open to pleasure . . . When a Sensual says they feel comfortable, that translates to "I'm turned on *now!*" When they are finally open to pleasure, you might see them breathing more deeply, or even moaning while tasting food or being touched.

Here's a list of turn-ons for a Sensual:

» A beautiful setting to make love in
» Helping them deeply relax
» Their whole body being touched
» Slow, connected, contouring touch to the curves and crevices of their skin
» Wonderful smells that delight them

» A musical soundtrack that drops them into their body
» Romantic contexts (think romantic movie scenes, dim lights, candles, moonlight, and warm cuddly nests to curl up in)
» Their favorite flowers
» Cleaning being done (and done well) for them
» Massages and spa time
» Vacation sex
» Getting things marked off their to-do list
» Someone taking the time to make things "just right" for them
» Lip balm
» Helping them feel like you want to take care of their needs instead of treating them as a burden or something too demanding
» Chocolate! Or other things they really enjoy eating.
» Hot baths or, better yet, a hot tub in a luxurious location where they can just be and relax

The environment they are in can really make or break a Sensual's turn-on. Having the right mindset and a beautiful setting are key to arousal for this Blueprint Type.

One of the biggest turn-ons for the Sensual is touch that follows the contours of their body and helps them relax more deeply. Add delicious-smelling oils that are warmed before they are applied, and you have a recipe for higher arousal. Sensuals love having time to luxuriate in touch without any pressure to move on to the main event. They want touch that allows the mystery of what's going to happen next to unfold organically.

The Sensual's Superpowers

Sensuals have many gifts, and when fully developed in their Superpowers, they are orgasmic wonderlands!

Embody It: Discovering the Sensual's Sweet Spot

Sensuals bring beauty to the erotic experience, and they are dazzled when you bring a beautiful, erotic experience to them.

To do this, you need to start thinking like a Sensual. That may be a difficult task, so I'm providing you with some questions to ask your Sensual lover.

To seduce a Sensual into your erotic world, you need to create a space where they feel totally relaxed and pampered. When you create this space, make sure you've paid attention to all five senses.

Ask your lover:

"What distracts you most during sex?"

"What are some tastes I can bring·to you? Would you like chocolates, fruit, or cheese? What about flavored edible lubricants?" (Find the nontoxic brands.)

"Do you like candles, flowers, dim lighting? What would please your eyes?"

"What sounds/music brings you the most pleasure?" Make sure to turn off your phone, or even put earbuds in your Sensual's ears, so they can be immersed in the soundscape without interruption. Make them a playlist they will never forget.

"What sensations do you love the most? Are you open to exploring what sensations might turn you on, like fur, contouring massage, silks, oils?"

Are all distractions put away? Have you paid attention to the details? How is your breath? Did you cut/file your fingernails? Have you showered, and are you smelling yummy?

And finally, what can you do to make sure your Sensual lover is deeply relaxed?

Take your time, and make sure not to rush! Sensuals love to relish relaxation.

From this starting point, you can slide into foreplay. Again—don't rush it! Simply let yourself be in the wonderful sensation of not knowing what's going to come next.

Like their turn-ons, the Sensual's Superpowers involve all the senses. When these Superpowers are fully unleashed, a Sensual can become so highly orgasmic that simple things, like the taste of chocolate, can make them weep in ecstasy.

Here are some common Sensual Superpowers:

» Orgasms arising from the senses being ignited
» Experiencing nongenital orgasms on a crevice of the body (for example, between the fingers)
» Full-body orgasms that shudder through every inch of them
» Deep and glorious surrender in their bodies
» Creating amazing spaces—they bring the beauty to any erotic experience
» Attention to all the details that make a difference

Sensuals have some amazing pathways to orgasm that don't involve the genitals at all (although genitals can certainly come to the party—they just aren't the guests of honor).

Sensuals can have orgasms just from eating something delicious (yes!). They'll frequently moan or do a happy dance while eating great food. That's a telltale sign someone has a strong Sensual component. It's fun to see. They may not even be aware they're moaning while they're doing it!

Embody It: Giving Yourself a Contouring Massage

If you are a Sensual, you can spend time each day giving yourself contouring touch while you apply lotion or oils to your body.

In Ayurveda, one of the oldest healing sciences from India, they use a daily oil massage called abhyanga. You get specific oils for your dosha (your individual Ayurvedic health blueprint) and massage them gently in circles over your joints. These oils are delicious, and sure to feed any Sensual. If you have a high Sensual Blueprint, include oil massages in your daily practice as you start your day. You can make this pleasure practice a habit, just like brushing your teeth!

If you're more of a lotion person, take time to contour your hands to your body as you apply it. Feel each delicious curve and crevice. Be mindful of how you are applying the lotion, and take deep breaths as your body meets the sensations of your hands gliding over your curves.

And, of course, if you have a partner, you can have them give you a ten-, sixty-, or ninety-minute contouring touch massage that consists of long, slow strokes with oil or lotion, where their hands contour themselves to your curves and kneed your muscles.

And while we're on the topic of orgasms: Sensuals can orgasm just about anywhere on the body. If you haven't taken the time to explore all the creases and crevices on a body, now's the time to get familiar with them! Try licking and touching behind the knees or going down on a Sensual's armpit (make sure they feel everything is clean and smells good so they're comfortable first).

When a Sensual can let go of their biggest challenge—getting caught up in their own head—they can move deeply into embodiment. When they are fully in their body, they can surrender to all the delicious waves of pleasure moving through it. They can go deep into a realm of experience where there's nothing to do, nothing to strive for, and nothing to change. They become united with the sensory experience, where the sensation and the person experiencing that sensation are one. This Superpower is one that can have a Sensual moaning and writhing in pleasure for hours, waving through orgasm after orgasm!

So Your Lover Is a Sensual . . .

If your lover is a Sensual, it can be so lovely for them to experience that you are slowing down and allowing things to organically unfold. Do your best to take any pressure to perform off their shoulders.

What could you do today to cross off a few items on their checklist? (Yes, this is some serious foreplay for a Sensual!)

I highly recommend that you discover romantic music that invites them to move their bodies. Make a playlist that you can listen to during lovemaking. Send them a song during the day that has lyrics about love (Sensuals love romantic contexts) or that is meaningful for your relationship.

One of my lovers of twenty years sent me a song recently that made my heart soar. The lyrics summed up our relationship in just four minutes.

Embody It: Owning Your Sensual Artistry

If you are Sensual, it's time that you own your sensual artistry!

Give yourself a budget and go shopping for delicious things that excite and ignite your erotic nature.

For the sense of touch, maybe buy some faux fur rugs for your bedroom, or some satin or linen sheets for your bed! Are there sensual sex toys you could add to your collection, like fur mitts, for example?

When thinking about smell, buy some new scents that just feel scrumptious when they're wafting through your home. Perhaps this is some incense, essential oils, or herbs you can burn.

For your sense of sight, bring some decorative pillows, live plants, or fresh flowers into your space. Adding art to your home can be a great way to delight your eyes.

When incorporating taste, what foods or flavors could you bring home to explore? Are there flavored lubricants you could add to your sexy play kit?

Maybe it's time to invest in that new speaker system so you can delight in sounds and music as you make love!

What are some simple things you can do today to fully own your love of detail and your ability to bring beauty into your erotic life?

You're one of the few things that I'm sure of . . . played from my speakers, and my body instantly responded in turn-on as tears ran down my cheeks. Music and romantic lyrics have that kind of power.

What can you do to light up all your lover's senses tonight? Is it having a great meal together? Or going dancing? How about giving them a long, slow massage without the agenda of getting to sex afterward?

Where to Begin If You Are Sensual

If you are Sensual and you want to fully develop in all your Superpowers, it's important to know which things help you to relax the most. And if you have a lover (or lovers), be sure to communicate these discoveries to them.

One of the most effective tools we have seen for Sensuals is the use of "toggles."

Toggles are an action or practice that helps you transition between your busy life and the erotic realms where you can just surrender and let go.

Here are a few toggles that many Sensuals love:

» Take ten to fifteen minutes to do some deep, slow breathing.

» Create a few anchor songs that remind you of your erotic nature and slowly move to them.

» Get a massage therapist to come to your house and rub you down.

» Take a long bath, steam shower, or even a cold shower/cold plunge.

» Put away all distractions and finish up a task you've been working on.

» Slow dance with a lover.

» Self-pleasure before your lover comes over/comes home.

» Hum and/or sing.

» Do some mindful meditation.

» Roll around naked on a faux fur rug.

» Take a nap.

» Make arrangements so there won't be any kids in the house before, during, and after lovemaking.

» Put on clothing made of silk or faux fur.

Journal Quickie: Your Sensual Toggles

Take a moment to journal about things that would help you transition more fully from a hectic day into your Sensual erotic world. You can use this prompt, then write down any ideas that come.

Prompt: Tell me something that would help you feel ready for sex.

Journal an unedited stream of thought for at least fifteen minutes.

Now you have a list of things that can help you to toggle into the realm of the erotic. Do these things before making love, either with yourself or with a partner.

For some of you, this Sensual world may very likely feel way too slow. You may be one of the many who is turned on and ready to go 24-7! If your pilot light never goes out, your tank is full, and you're always ready to accelerate from zero to sixty in seconds, I won't make you wait any longer.

Let's get it on!

CHAPTER NINE

the sexual

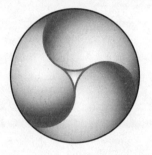

Sex is the driving force on the planet. We should
embrace it, not see it as the enemy.

—HUGH HEFNER

You Might Be a Sexual Blueprint If . . .

» You bring the fun to sex. Sex is simple and easy. Arousal, orgasm, and/or ejaculation are all easily attainable.

» You're turned on by naked bodies, genitals, direct genital touch, overtly erotic sounds, imagery, and videos.

» You have sex to feel more relaxed.

» Having sex makes you feel seen, honored, loved, and desired. If sex is not happening regularly, something feels wrong.

» When you're unable to act on it, your desire can sometimes feel like physical pain or intense anxiety.

» You can be very focused on the goal of reaching orgasm.

» You've been shamed or judged for your voracious desire for sex or your overt expressions of sexuality, especially if you're a woman who is a Sexual; you may have been slut-shamed during your life and tamped down your high libido in an effort to conform.

» You don't understand why everyone else makes sex so complicated. Setting up a romantic environment is a hassle, doing all that rope-tie stuff is boring, and eye-gazing and breathing together is weird.

» You hear from your lover(s) that they feel objectified and need more than just intercourse to be satisfied.

» You are sometimes resistant to opportunities to expand your erotic intelligence.

Heads up, sexy language ahead! If you're not a Sexual Blueprint Type, prepare for some uncensored explicit talk about sex.

Welcome to the Sexual Blueprint, where we love sex (fucking, humping, licking, sucking), and we love genitals (dicks, clits, pussies, balls), and we love orgasms (cumming, squirting, getting off, ejaculating)!

It's rare that I get the opportunity to really speak to Sexuals. Due to censorship, or more conservative teaching environments, it's sometimes challenging to really give this Blueprint what it loves most when I'm teaching. Get ready, because this chapter is giving it to you hot!

The Sexual Shadows

"I want him inside of me. I want orgasms multiple times a day. I crave him. Jaiya, I think about sex all the time. I count the days that go by when we didn't have sex. To say I am frustrated is an understatement. We're married, doesn't that mean we owe each other sex?" Julia's voice demonstrated her frustration and anger over not getting the amount of sex she craved.

She wanted sex. She wanted a lot of it. She wanted it now.

She didn't need foreplay or a beautiful environment.

She just wanted to be penetrated, to have him inside her.

"It's like you're a juicy grape withering on the vine, no one coming to pluck you and eat you," I said, giving her empathy through an analogy. I could empathize with her because I had been in a similar situation with Ian.

She nodded in agreement. "He wants to do all these things I just don't want to do. If he's not giving me sex, why should I bother?" she said, exasperated.

The challenge was that Julia wasn't patient when it came to feeding the erotic needs of her husband of five years. When a Sexual is starving, the last thing they want to do is to create a sexy environment or a playlist or do some big kinky scene.

Julia didn't want to take that time. She wanted to fuck and be fucked. And she wanted to reach climax!

"I know I shouldn't have done this, but the other day I walked into the bedroom, and I literally said, 'Let's fuck right now, I can't stand this any longer!'" she admitted. Her husband was a clear Sensual, so this behavior was horrible foreplay for him because pressure killed his turn-on.

The sad part was that Julia was really missing the delicious journey she and her husband could be having together. All she was focused on was getting to it and achieving the end goal of intercourse and orgasm that she craved like oxygen.

Over time, the frustration turned to judgment and resentment in their relationship. She couldn't understand what in the world was wrong with him. She was sexy, he even told her how attractive she was to him. When they had sex, it was great! They would always have orgasms, so what was the problem with him?

Julia would also get frustrated because she wanted certainty that they were going to have penetration and that she was going to have an orgasm.

"Last night he said it to me again—'Let's just see how this unfolds.' I don't want to see how it's going to unfold, I want to know that he is going to fuck me!" She was close to pounding her fists in her lap; they were clenched as much as her jaw, she was so upset.

Julia's story perfectly matches the Shadow side of the Sexual.

I could feel her pain. Can you?

Luckily (though regrettably), I've been in her shoes, so I knew I could help if she and her husband were willing. Ian and I had found an amazing solution to this challenge by overlapping my Sexual Blueprint and his Kinky Blueprint.

Julia had a lot of Sexual Shadows and she thought for sure that something was wrong with her husband. "I mean, aren't all cisgender men supposed to want sex all the time?" she asked me. I explained how my colleagues and I discovered that not all cis men are Sexuals, and that it's wrong to assume they are.

I hear the Shadows of the Sexual so often that I'm not surprised at all when a new client brings them to me. I know right away that they're in the Sexual Shadow.

Here are some Shadow statements that I hear frequently:

» "I can't get enough sex."
» "I just want to get to the penetration."
» "I need certainty that we're going to have sex and orgasms."
» "I don't understand what's wrong with my lover."
» "Why aren't we having sex all the time?"
» "I feel bad that I can't control my sexual needs."
» "Why is my partner so complex? Sex is easy—it shouldn't require all this preparation and complication."
» "Can't we just get to it, already?"
» "Nothing is wrong with our sex life; we're having orgasms, so it's fine."
» "We're married, so it's my partner's obligation—that's what marriage is, right?"

You see, for a Sexual, sex is like food, air, or water. It isn't just something they like to do—it's something they *need*.

But with such a strong need, they can get deeply frustrated and angry and impatient when that need isn't met. They don't understand lovers whose Blueprint differs from their own.

THE TOXIC SEXUAL

Sexuals in the Shadow, with unprocessed anger and frustration, can go overboard with unwanted advances and a lack of understanding or honoring of consent and boundaries. This is a very unhealthy and toxic version of a Sexual Type who just wants to take what they want, without regard for the other human being(s) involved.

Other people can become nonconsensual objects for meeting the Sexual's needs.

It can be difficult for those who are not Sexually Blueprinted to understand just how powerful this drive for sex and need for orgasm can be for the Sexual Type. Sex is essential to them as living beings—and can feel like a matter of life or death. Imagine what happens when you go without air for too long, and you'll have a good idea of the pain some Sexual Blueprints endure. This is not to excuse toxic or nonconsensual behavior by Sexuals, but to bring awareness to where this behavior stems from.

For a Sexual who is not having sex, the level of internal pain can feel like the pressure in a champagne bottle being endlessly shaken with the cork still in place. This level of tension and the need to have it relieved can have the partner of a Sexual Type feel like a piece of meat—there to be consumed and the leftovers disposed of after the feast is complete.

Being used like this by the Sexual can build resentment in the partner's mind and body. They may close off to their Sexual lover because they've had months or years of having their boundaries crossed just to meet their partner's need. The Sexual is unconscious to this, especially when there is assumed consent in a relationship. They often have no idea anything is wrong, and feel slighted when they find out their behavior makes their partner feel used or unsafe. The Sexual may also be troubled to learn that their partner finds their sex life unfulfilling.

Unfortunately, I see this in our practice far too often.

A lot of communication and healing must take place before the Sexual can expect to get their needs met, because by the time they've come to see me, the non-Sexual person has shut down their sexuality entirely.

This drive toward releasing sexual tension and the goal of orgasm and ejaculation leads to one of the Sexual's other big Shadows . . .

MISSING OUT ON THE EROTIC JOURNEY

Sexuals in the Shadow can miss the erotic journey because they're too focused on the end destination of orgasm or goal of sex.

I hear so often from Sexuals that they're resistant to feeding their partner's Erotic Blueprint because they just want to get what *they* want. They don't understand that by taking the time to explore the journey and allow things to unfold more organically, they'll have a much more satisfying experience with their lover(s).

Sexuals are usually thinking a hundred steps ahead of all the other Blueprints, and that's part of the reason they're so frustrated. They just want to get to the end, because that hot, juicy orgasm and ejaculation is what allows them to relax, helps them feel connected and alive, and boosts their confidence.

SEX IS ALWAYS ON THE BRAIN

Sexuals in the Shadow often complain that they can't understand why anything is wrong with the relationship or with their approach to sex. They often feel blindsided when a lover shares that they're dissatisfied with their sex life.

If there's penetration and orgasms, why would anyone need to work on improving their sex life? Right? Sexuals don't see that there's more to the sexual experience than having an orgasm or having penetrative-style sex.

Sexuals think about sexual intercourse and orgasms more frequently than any other Erotic Blueprint. They usually have the highest libidos and want sex more frequently, too.

But what happens when their lover's libido doesn't match theirs?

The brutal part of this Shadow is that Sexuals will blame their lover and will often, in anger and frustration, state that something must be wrong with their partner.

Pleasure First: Guided Fantasy

Place your dominant hand on your genitals and notice the feeling of your genitals beneath your hand.

Think about someone you would like to fuck.

Notice what happens beneath your hand.

With your hand on your genitals, think about someone sexy, and begin to make circles over your genitals.

Notice what happens beneath your hand.

Now, begin to contract and relax your pelvic floor muscles.

Notice what happens beneath your hand.

With your hand on your genitals, continue thinking about someone sexy, making circles over your genitals, and contracting and relaxing your pelvic floor muscles. Exhale as you contract your pelvic floor, and inhale as you relax.

Notice what happens beneath your hand.

Now just touch your genitals however you like—until you're satisfied!

It's easy for a Sexual to feel righteous in this way because we live in a culture that predominately says great sex falls in the Sexual Blueprint. So if a person isn't easily aroused or isn't having mind-blowing orgasms all the time, that must mean they're broken and wrong. But as you're learning in this book, many people do not live in the Sexual Blueprint.

HOW MUCH SEX IS TOO MUCH SEX?

Some Sexuals may wonder if they have a "sex addiction." It can become a distressing Shadow. From the Erotic Blueprint perspective, a Sexual may receive this label from a partner who is a different Erotic Blueprint. And that's really painful. Some Sexuals may feel this label fits if it seems like they aren't getting their sexual needs met and/or if they consistently want more sexual intercourse than their partner.

Since sex is a natural and pleasurable part of life, this labeling can be damaging, and wound a person's sexuality, functioning, and relationships.

In relationships, the "sex addict" label tends to be placed on the person who wants more intercourse than their partner. Some say the label is an excuse used by those who refuse to accept responsibility for their sexual choices. Others use the description to pass moral judgment on those whose sex lives (or pornography use) doesn't fit with societal norms or personal beliefs.

We're here to understand a person's erotic needs with openness, love, and compassion, not to judge each other or assign labels that do more harm than good.

Sex addiction is not a clinical diagnosis. In fact, it was rejected from the latest version of the *DSM* (*Diagnostic and Statistical Manual of Mental Disorders*). However, some people may experience out-of-control sexual behaviors that cause them distress.

According to the World Health Organization (WHO), compulsive sexual behavior disorder is diagnosed when a person's sexual impulses and urges are so intense, they are unable to control their behavior. Various sexual activities become the person's primary focus in life, even if they aren't receiving any pleasure from those behaviors. Additionally, they neglect other important aspects of their life, resulting in negative consequences.

So how much sex is too much sex? There's no right answer. It's a balance between your needs and your partner's needs. It's up to you as an individual. The "right" amount of sex is whatever amount feels right for you, as long as it's pleasurable to you and not hurting anyone else. Only you know what's best.

LIMITED DEFINITION OF SEX

Sexuals define successful sex as intercourse, with hard cocks and/or wet pussies involved, that ends with a climax.

So if erections aren't present, the whole experiment is a failure.

If there isn't wetness, something must be wrong.

If they don't have an orgasm, well, that's another failure.

Phil was diagnosed with prostate cancer, and after the removal of his prostate, he could no longer achieve erections. Due to his limited definition of sex and this big change in his sexual function, he was certain his sexual life was over for good. His wife, however, longed for physical and intimate connection with Phil. So they came to see me.

Phil was unaware that there was a Sensual or Energetic realm that he could learn to make love in. I taught Phil how to expand his viewpoints on what made sex great by tapping into the world of Energetic sex.

"I just had the most amazing orgasm!" he exclaimed to me. "I thought sex was over for me and Deb. But now, wow, there's a whole world I didn't even know I was missing. My body was in so much pleasure, and I didn't even need an erection. It was the best sex we've ever had!" He was over the moon after this newfound experience, one he'd never imagined because he'd limited his understanding of sex to physical penetration.

Before we move on to all the wonderful aspects of the Sexual and all the awesome things that turn them on, I need to address an interesting phenomenon that happens with this Blueprint.

THE SEXUAL MASK

Over my thirty years of practice, I've seen so many people put on what I call a "sexual mask" because they think that's how they're supposed to be if they are a healthy sexual being. When someone takes on living as if this Blueprint is their Primary Blueprint, whether because of shame or because they don't know any other way to be, that is their sexual mask.

Embody It: A Sexual's Sweet Spot

Bring some creativity into your play with a Sexual partner by making small gestures that feed their Blueprint:

» Greet them by touching their genitals and giving them appreciation.

» Make dinner with nothing but an apron on.

» Striptease for them.

» Give them spontaneous oral sex.

» Go shopping for sex toys together, either online or by visiting a novelties store.

» Allow them to put a vibrator directly on your genitals or stimulate you in some other way until you orgasm.

» Tell them which night you're going to have sex with them— and then make sure to follow through.

» Hump each other.

» Watch porn or read erotica together.

These can all be fun and creative ways to turn on a Sexual lover!

I once had a client who was trying to be like "all the other guys." He had done course after course on sex, tried sleeping with sex workers, taken performance-enhancing drugs, and hung out in bars in order to be what he thought a man should be sexually. By the time he came to me, it seemed like nothing that "should" turn him on did, and he had so much self-hatred.

I was his last resort.

I quickly discovered that he was clearly not a Sexual. He was just trying to fit himself into the Sexual Blueprint because he didn't know any other way to be.

In the Netflix series *Sex, Love & Goop*, you (spoiler alert!) see Damon go through this transformation as well. As a big, masculine man, he thought he needed to be a certain way, and all he knew from his peers and how he grew up was the Sexual Blueprint, so he thought for sure he was Sexual, and he tried acting as such. But as tears rolled down his face and he started to have energetic orgasms during one of our table sessions, everyone could clearly see that the Sexual Blueprint was not responsible for his most intense turn-on.

SEXUAL SHAME

One last Shadow of the Sexual Type, especially for those of us with vulvas, is sexual shame.

Women are especially shamed for our sexual nature. We're sluts or whores if we love, crave, and seek out sexual connections. This can lead many of us to shut down our sexuality. We stop expressing who we are as erotic beings and start hiding and judging ourselves. Slut-shaming needs to come to an end. It's time for women—especially women who are Sexuals—to claim their erotic empowerment and evolution by releasing shame.

Brené Brown, researcher, speaker, and author on topics such as shame, has an amazing definition that helps us distinguish between guilt and shame. She says that guilt is when we say to ourselves, "I've done something wrong or bad." And shame is when we say to ourselves, "I am bad."

How do you talk to yourself about your sexuality? Do you tell yourself that you are bad or wrong for your sexual desires? It might be time to do some unraveling and healing of shame about who you are.

Sex is natural. Babies in the womb stimulate their own genitals. We are born with desire.

Sex is how we all got here.

It's time to stop shaming our nature and instead celebrate our Sexual turn-ons.

The Sexual's Turn-Ons

Sexuals are turned on by what we as a culture stereotypically think of as sex.

Current media is shifting in some small part to reflect a wider variety of sexual experiences. For decades, however, mainstream media, as well as internet porn, has solely showcased the sexual narrative of the white heterosexual couple—one with a penis and the other with a vagina—who have sex until ejaculation or orgasm. The most ideal depiction is a photo finish of simultaneous orgasm, which is even less realistic. If it's a romantic narrative, the couple gets married and they live happily ever after!

But healthy, amazing sex happens between people of all races and consenting ages, all genders and sexual orientations. The erotic realm is available to everyone.

Although a Sexual's approach to sex looks very simple (which can be one of the Superpowers that we'll discuss later), Sexuals, when fully expressed, have a depth of turn-on and a wider variety of turn-on than what this cultural narrative portrays. Simply put, Sexuals don't just love penetration, orgasms, and nudity; they also love deep connection and deep bonding.

Sexuals are turned on by:

» Nudity

» Direct genital stimulation and rubbing

» Certainty that they are going to have sex and orgasms

» Penetration

» Orgasms

» Simplicity

» Dressing provocatively or in very sexy clothing

» Pornography and other visuals

» Frequent sex

» Oral sex

» Anal sex

» Bodily fluids

» Masturbation

» Quickies

» Spontaneity

» Frequency

» Swinging or nonmonogamy

» Use of vibrators, dildos, and other directly sexual sex toys

» Erotic imagery

Because of their high sex drive, Sexuals may choose ways of being in relationships that are not traditional. For example, they may be turned on by practicing nonmonogamy or participating in swinger lifestyles. Ian and I express in nontraditional orientations and relationship styles. Ian currently identifies as being bisexual, and I identify as pansexual (I like it all). We're both polyamorous, which is a nonmonogamous relationship style.

Being poly, I can more fully express my pansexual nature and feed all my Erotic Blueprint desires. This doesn't mean that if you are Sexual, you must be this way, too. It simply means that we all get to express our individual sexuality in various ways depending on our Erotic Blueprint, sexual orientation, gender identity, gender expression, and relationship style.

But I digress.

Let's get back to Sexuals and what sparks their turn-on.

Simply put, Sexuals love sex. They love to have it often. And not just sex with another person (or persons)—they like sex with themselves, too.

Self-pleasure is a way for Sexuals to relieve tension and take pressure off their partners, who may not have the same drive or desire around sexual intercourse. Sexuals are very visual, so having a healthy relationship with pornography can be a big turn-on for them. It's important not to shame yourself (or others) if you love to self-pleasure while viewing erotica.

The Sexual's Superpowers

Kyle had been working with me for three years and had fully owned who he was erotically. Being a primary Sexual, he dealt with a lot of tension around his desires for sexual intercourse and where to put all that sexual energy!

"I used to think my sexuality was a curse I had to get rid of," said Kyle. "But now"—he smiled at me with a look of knowing—"now I feel so grateful that I am who I am."

I loved watching him expand fully into his Superpowers and own himself so confidently. I loved how healthy he's become in his expression and how he's embraced his Superpowers.

Just like all the other Blueprints, Sexuals have some amazing abilities, and when brought out of the Shadow, they are truly wonderful lovers.

Here's a quick look at some of the Sexual's Superpowers:
- » Shameless, freely expressed sexuality that gives others permission to be sexual, too!
- » Quick arousal time; they're usually walking around aroused, so it doesn't take much!
- » Erotic ease and simplicity, with access to emotional depth
- » Bring the joy and fun to erotic experiences
- » Can become deeply relaxed during sex
- » Sex is a mood booster and a tool for feeling like everything is going right in their world.

It's so awesome that in terms of arousability, Sexuals can go from zero to sixty in seconds. Because they're often thinking about sex and wondering when they'll have sex next, their pilot light is always on. And when that turn-on is channeled appropriately, it can become fuel for greater energy levels, creativity, and fullness of living.

Sexuals bring the joy and the fun to sex! It doesn't have to be so serious. Let's play!

To a Sexual, sex is a magical, fulfilling, and satisfying way to spend time together. Getting off is great! Why wouldn't everyone want to do it as much as possible?

This is something some of the other Blueprints could learn from them. Sexuals give us all permission.

When Sexuals have sex and orgasms, they feel relaxed; they feel like everything is right in the world. Sexuals have sex to relax, whereas Sensuals need to relax before they have sex. This is a key fact when thinking about Blueprint Compatibility, which I'll cover later in this book!

SIMPLICITY AND DEPTH

Kyle brought to my awareness how Sexuals in our community were perceived as too simple and lacking depth. But simple doesn't mean without depth. Just because someone is easily turned on and loves sex doesn't mean they can't create deep and intimate bonds or want a beautiful connection with those they make love with.

As a matter of fact, for many Sexuals, sex equals love. And not having sex with your Sexual partner or not showing your desire for them can feel to them as if you don't love them, even if that's not true for you.

Sex and love can be complicated for any Blueprint, but especially so for a Sexual.

So Your Lover Is a Sexual . . .

If you have someone who is a Sexual Type in your life, feeding them is rather simple: Just have sex with them. Cook dinner naked or topless. Allow them to touch you sexually. Have a weekly oral sex night. It really can be that simple.

However, if you've spent weeks, months, or years overriding your boundaries to satisfy their drive for intercourse, or your Blueprint needs and desires have been overlooked in deference to theirs, you may have built up resistance—or even resentment.

Every advance has become unwanted, because you do not feel seen by or perhaps don't even feel safe with your Sexual partner. Perhaps you're uncomfortable with oral sex, or your desire for sex is much lower than your lover's and you can't keep pace with them.

Working through your own resistance to integrate the Sexual Blueprint is a challenge for many. Before you try these practices with your Sexual partner, make sure you're ready and willing.

Establishing your boundaries and having them honored is an essential first step. For example, let your Sexual lover know that just because you are touching their genitals doesn't mean you are going to have intercourse. Remember, Sexuals love certainty. Give certainty of what will and won't happen, and they can relax more into the fun of the game.

If your lover is a Sexual, it's time to look at all the places where you can acknowledge, accept, and appreciate who they are a lot more than you have in the past. And then to give it to them—directly, and usually with genital stimulation. Seriously.

I asked a group of Sexuals in our community what would make them feel the most appreciated, and almost all of them said they would love to be greeted with touch to their genitals while being told how much they are appreciated.

Embody It: Self-Pleasure Practice

Let's take your masturbation to the next level with this self-pleasure practice!

What if, for the next five days, you mindfully used your daily masturbation to expand more deeply into a healthy sexual expression?

Try this! Each day, set aside thirty minutes or more to really focus on your self-pleasure.

DAY ONE: What is your normal way of pleasuring yourself? Begin by touching yourself the way you normally do during self-pleasure; this is to get a baseline. Do this for ten minutes, but do not come to climax.

For the next ten minutes, add conscious breathing. Inhale and exhale through your mouth. Breath increases arousal. Keep breathing like this for the rest of the session while you touch yourself as you normally do.

For the last ten minutes, add fantasy or visualization. Imagine penetrating or being penetrated. What if a lover was going down on you? Use the tool of visualization to further enhance your experience.

DAY TWO: You will need to have a vibrator to play with on day two. It doesn't matter if you are cock-bodied or vulva-bodied to play with a vibrator.

Begin by touching yourself, adding the conscious breathing from day one, then some visualization. You're combining all three for the first ten minutes of this practice.

For the next ten minutes, add the vibrator, touching it to a nongenital part of your body, though you can tease over your genital area. I recommend placing the vibrator on your inner thighs, pubic bone, perineum, and/or chest.

In the final ten minutes, begin to give more genital focus, but make sure you don't climax until the time is up. And remember to keep using the tools of breath and visualization in your practice.

DAY THREE: Take the first ten minutes to find something visually stimulating, such as an erotic still photo or a video.

For the next twenty minutes, look at this visual while you pleasure yourself. Make sure you stay present and mindful of what you're doing physically, and don't forget to breathe. Joseph Kramer, the creator of Sexological Bodywork and one of my mentors, calls this "porn yoga."

DAY FOUR: Take off all your clothing. Stand naked in front of a mirror. Take the first five minutes just to gaze at your naked body. Take the next five minutes to gaze specifically at your genitals.

Now watch yourself in your self-pleasure practice. You can close your eyes for a moment but really gaze at yourself as you're self-pleasuring. You can use your vibrator and your breath, but you are the visualization itself. Do this for the next fifteen minutes.

For the last five minutes, bring yourself to climax and see if you can keep your eyes open to watch yourself have an orgasm.

DAY FIVE: Now it's time to celebrate. Do a longer session—I recommend at least an hour—and put together some of the favorite things that you discovered over the past four days.

Sexuals don't usually get what they crave because their lovers are afraid that they will be expected to have intercourse. So, Sexuals, if you want delicious greetings like this, you need to let go of the expectation that it means your partner is available for penetration.

Where to Begin If You Are a Sexual

If you are Sexual and you're interested in expanding into new territory and fully developing your own Blueprint, I have two recommendations.

1. FEED YOURSELF

Most Sexuals could use more time getting their erotic needs met. How can you get fed?

Could you start a self-pleasure practice, like the one described earlier in this chapter? Could you have a conversation with your partner about how they could be more sexual with you? What are some healthy, consensual ways you could express your sexuality that create a feeling of fulfillment for you?

Look at the list of ways that Sexuals love being turned on and make your own list of ways you can feel more fulfilled. For example, maybe you love the suggestion to have your lover greet you each day by placing a hand on your genitals and sharing how much they love and appreciate you.

2. PATIENCE, UNDERSTANDING, AND LEARNING

The biggest Shadow for the Sexual, which undercuts their ability to forge satisfying sexual partnerships, is that they don't quite understand or have patience for the pleasures that feed the other Erotic Blueprints.

If your Primary Blueprint is the Sexual, but your partner's isn't, this can be a very big problem for you.

Journal Quickie: Feed Me!

I know that for most Sexuals, journaling about sex isn't their favorite activity. But maybe you could enhance this journal exercise by having someone go down on you while you write.

Don't get too distracted—you still need to write!

Take some time to make a list of all the things you feel would feed you sexually. Don't limit yourself based on what you think your partner would be okay with (or not). Go for it. Go wild! Uncensored!

If you have a lover, share some of the things on your list with them.

"Ugh! Why do we need to do all that unnecessary stuff? Sex is simple. I don't have time for all these complications," you might say. This attitude can leave your lover feeling unseen, unfulfilled, and, in some cases, abused. How can you learn more about what turns them on?

Are you willing to try some of those things combined with your own Sexual expressions?

For example, could you touch your genitals in a way that is erotic and pleasing and at the same time put on some Sensual music? Maybe this still doesn't do it for you, but at least you can understand that it might do it for someone else, and that opens a big door for mutual satisfaction.

You are likely very visual in your eroticism. You may learn best by watching. (And no, porn is not a very good teacher, but it can be great for arousal.)

I alluded earlier to Ian and I finding a super-hot solution to my desire to have more intercourse and genital play and his lack of spontaneous interest or initiation. This solution came about by combining the Sexual and Kinky Blueprints.

Well, this next chapter we're going to get Kinky.

Discovering Ian's kink and learning how to feed it along with my Sexual Blueprint was exactly what set him on fire. He was turned on by the power dynamic, and I was getting exactly what I needed.

So behave yourself [*Jaiya gets out her whip*], and read on NOW!

If you're good, you might just get a naughty pleasure treat!

CHAPTER TEN

the kinky

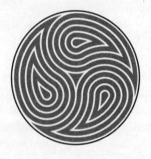

I like your pants around your feet
And I like the dirt that's on your knees
And I like the way you still say please
While you're looking up at me.

—"FIGURED YOU OUT" BY NICKELBACK

You Might Be a Kinky Blueprint If . . .

» You are turned on by thinking of or doing things you think are taboo, think you shouldn't do, or think are naughty or edgy.

» You love psychological power games of control and surrender, dominance and submission.

» You are very creative in your erotic play, setting up scenes and scenarios, role play, or character play.

» You love intense sensation or physically edgy play, receiving or giving spanks and scratches, hair pulling, flogging, constriction, choking, or being choked.

» You love being physically restrained or restraining another person with ropes, straps, cuffs, or other forms of constriction.

» It's possible for you to reach such heightened states of turn-on that you can orgasm without even being touched.

» You have developed the skills to create consent agreements before you play with a lover, clearly articulating your needs and desires and declaring what's allowed and what's not.

» Respecting boundaries has become part of your emotional and erotic practice with yourself and with other people.

» You may experience shame because of what naturally turns you on, thinking it is wrong or that you are weird or broken because of your desires.

» You may find yourself getting stuck in a pattern of taboo eroticism that becomes your only route to turn-on. You may feel constrained by this limitation.

You may have fears and judgments about kinky sex.

I know I did.

Earlier in my life, when I was living in my Energetic Shadow, believing that spiritual sexuality was the only way people should be having sex, I judged kinky people. Long ago, I cried over one of my lover's bruises, unable to comprehend why someone would, or could, enjoy this kind of pleasure.

Because of these judgments and my lack of understanding around kinky sexual expression, I didn't even include it as one of the Blueprint Types until several months after I discovered the Blueprints.

You may also have an image in your mind that kinky sex is full of black leather, bondage, pain, and submission. Kink can include all of that . . . but the world of kink is vast, and the creativity available within the realms of kink is endless.

Kink means whatever is taboo for you, and it's way more varied than you might think. And "taboo" itself means different things to different people. I've had clients who perceive sex outside of the missionary position as extra naughty, and this also fits into the realm of kinky sex.

You may be kinky and not even know it!

Are you leaning in with curiosity now?

Are you ready for more?

Say "please."

Louder—I can't hear you.

I like that. You're sooooo good. And I love it when you behave.

The Shadow Side of the Kinky

"Why am I so turned on by this?" Ian had a look of wonder on his face as I took the red rope and tied his hands to his feet. "Shhh . . . I didn't give you permission to speak!" I exclaimed, reminding him of our agreements. "You are not allowed to speak unless you ask permission to do so."

Pleasure First: Kitchen Kink

Let's explore some intense sensation.

My friend Jaeleen Bennis, creator of Bondassage, says that you can make anything a "pervertible"! Things in your kitchen make great kinky toys. Gather a fork, a spatula, or a wooden spoon. How about a whisk or a rubber band? Oooh, what about an ice cube or two?

Try tapping that spatula or wooden spoon lightly on your buttocks. Now tap harder, increasing the intensity. As you increase the intensity, where does it feel most pleasurable? Play with speed as well; what happens when you go faster, or slower, with more space and anticipation between taps? Try tapping in rhythm as if your booty is a drum available for a musician to play.

Oh, that ice cube on your neck! What happens when you let the cold contact your most sensitive skin? How can you more fully meet the intense sensation? (Hint: Breath and movement are both ways you can meet intensity more fully.)

What about that rubber band in your junk drawer? Snap it on your forearm. Give yourself a little sting.

Run a fork up your inner thigh. Want to get a little edgy? How about scraping a knife along your thigh? Don't puncture the skin, just feel the danger of the edge of the knife lightly scratching.

Keep playing with random objects around your kitchen and exploring the sensations they provide. Notice what is most pleasurable, and add it to your erotic play kit!

He stayed quiet and began to enjoy the feeling of the ropes on his skin.

I'd never seen an erection like the one he had in that moment. His arousal was through the roof, but it was obvious from his question that he still felt uneasy about the fact that he liked being tied up.

We were six and a half years into our relationship before I discovered that Ian's fastest path to arousal was through the Kinky Blueprint.

After years of suffering for lack of sexual connection in our relationship, I finally discovered that all I needed to do was lay the red ropes on the bed.

So how could a sex educator go for six years without knowing this about her partner?

One word: shame.

As I sit here writing, Ian and I are about to celebrate seventeen years together. It's been wonderful, and we've shared life to its fullest. A couple of years into our relationship, we had a child together. We now share a business together. We share a bed, we share our hardships, and we share our glories and celebrations.

He is my lifetime love and lover.

And yet it took him more than six years into our relationship to begin to come to terms with who he is as an erotic being and just how kinky (and queer) he is.

Each year, he owns more of his erotic expression. Each year, he peels away another layer of shame that comes along with his kinky truth. It's been so hot to watch him overcome this shame and claim his pleasure.

Shame can be overwhelming for a Kinky. Shame for being turned on by what is considered taboo. Shame for their desires. Shame for being who they are. And shame isn't the only Shadow side of the Kinky Blueprint.

Some of the common Shadows of the Kinky include:

» Shame for taboo turn-ons that restricts sexual expression
» Fear that turn-ons must mean something is wrong
  psychologically

» Turn-ons that get stuck and become dead ends

» Unconsciously playing out unhealed trauma in order to heal

» Putting yourself in unhealthy, unsafe situations due to lack of education

As we explored the corners of kinky play in our lovemaking, Ian would often struggle with his turn-ons. He wanted to understand why he was wired the way he was wired. We had both inherited a common and mistaken belief that Kinky desires must all arise from trauma. But Ian had no experience with sexual trauma in his personal life.

There's a myth that being kinky comes with a pathology. But that's so far from the truth.

Research shows that kinky people do not suffer from mental illness to a greater extent than the general population. Despite the increased visibility of kink practices in popular media, the stigma attached to the practice is still widespread, and misconceptions about kink practitioners are common. The incorrect assumption is that a person's desire to engage in kink is linked to an exposure to violence, past traumatic experiences, and mental health issues. But several major research studies have concluded that people who engage in and enjoy kink aren't more likely to have a history of trauma or mental illness.

Kink is also empowering to people who do have a history of trauma, and can help navigate past experiences of powerlessness, embarrassment, discomfort, and stress. Kink practices enable people to accept parts of themselves that are stigmatized. Kinky folks often use "scenes" to work through those feelings in a way that can feel therapeutic.

A 2018 study by Richard Sprott and Bren Hadcock of bisexual, pansexual, and queer kink participants found that kink activities can have many uses, including gender exploration and healing from shame and trauma related to sexual identity/orientation.

Anyone, no matter their Blueprint, can experience and be imprinted by a history of trauma and abuse, and I'm here to tell you there's nothing wrong with you if you are a Kinky Type. I'm also here to give you permission to enjoy this aspect of yourself, as long as your expression is safe and consensual.

As a matter of fact, studies have shown that people who are kinky, and have cultivated conscientious expressions of their kinky desires, usually have better communication skills, better understanding of consent and boundaries, and the ability to craft sexual experiences that are safe and healthy.

So why all the shame?

Well, any time we participate in something that feels outside the "norm" of the way we think we're "supposed" to be, there's an opportunity for us to say that we are flawed, or that something is wrong with us.

Anyone who's been part of a nondominant or marginalized community inherently understands what this is like. You start to feel shame about who you are, and you creatively hide who you are, for fear of being cast out, ostracized, or worse. Imagine living in a world where who you are, your being, your identity, is threatened.

Some of you reading this don't have to imagine it—you've lived it, or you're still living it.

In Ian's case, it has been a slow unfolding of his sexuality and of his realization that his Kinky parts do not have edges. As he dives more deeply into this area of play, he continues to discover more and more taboo things that turn him on.

On a personal and professional level, I am so thrilled each time he discovers more of himself through kink. And I'm grateful that he has love and support all around him to help him own and explore these turn-ons. As a leader, every time he comes out a bit more, he gives our entire community more permission to be who they are.

A SEXUAL GRAVEYARD: ONE ROUTE TO AROUSAL

We want you to have many ways in which you can be aroused and find sexual satisfaction. Instead of one route to your orgasm, what if you had thousands?

What happens, though, when a fantasy or a taboo turn-on becomes the only route to pleasure?

In my clinical experience, this once novel expression eventually becomes a rut, and then a grave. It forms a neural highway in your brain and cuts off other pathways to pleasure. And this can become distressing.

"I can't get turned on by anything else! I'll never find a woman who will understand this." Billie was sobbing in my office, in a lot of distress. "Seriously, there is nothing else that turns me on like this, and I can't admit it to anyone."

The "this" Billie was referring to was his desire to wear women's stockings. He not only had deep shame around this kink, which only made the turn-on higher by making it more taboo, he had fixated on wearing stockings during self-pleasure for over twenty years. His turn-on had become a grave. He had no access to other forms of arousal.

There was nothing wrong with his turn-on—wearing women's stockings can feel delicious and, for someone who identified as a man, kinky or taboo. But Billie had lost conscious choice over his own arousal; he could no longer connect to the wide variety of other turn-ons available to him. Compounded by his shame, the belief that no one could love him if they knew his secret desires had left him in a state of hopeless distress.

But what if a turn-on is so taboo that there isn't a healthy way to express it? For example, wanting to override the boundaries of others, causing physical harm to someone, or using hard and highly addictive drugs to enhance the sexual experience. Your desire for it may increase and become more deeply ingrained. The more ingrained it is, the higher the unhealthy turn-on becomes. The shame and hiding may increase, which then drives more craving.

I think many people can relate to this when it comes to attraction to someone we know isn't good for us. The sex is great! The attraction is irresistible! But we know it's a toxic relationship. Staying in that relationship is unhealthy, yet we keep going back for more and more. It's like a drug that we know is going to make us feel bad the next day and have a detrimental effect on our lives, yet we can't resist it.

However, if you have a primary taboo turn-on, healthy ways to experience and express it, and lovers in your life who don't desire more from you, then there's nothing wrong with a singular route to pleasure. Just stay alert so you'll be aware when this singular path to turn-on and satisfaction moves into the Shadow side.

Ending this self-fulfilling downward spiral requires shining a light into the Shadows, accepting that your desires are normal and finding ways to express them healthfully and consensually. If these feelings become so distressing that they prevent you from living your life or you feel like they are controlling you, it's time to get help. Talk to an expert who can support you.

THE SHADOW OF UNRESOLVED TRAUMA

Fortunately, the stigma around kinky play and kink lifestyle is dropping away. The American Psychiatric Association removed consensual BDSM (bondage and discipline, dominance and submission, sadism and masochism) and fetish play from the *DSM* in 2013. You can be a Kinky Type without having ever experienced traumatic sexual events—but if, in fact, you *have* experienced sexual trauma, I recommend that you take extra care in exploring this realm of sexuality.

Power games and intense physical sensation play can be part of this style of intimacy, and you may experience some triggering of your trauma as a result. Making sure you're aware of this and that you have skilled support to guide you through these triggers is strongly advised.

I have personal experience with this.

Ian and I dove into a 40/40 kink experiment while researching my book *Cuffed, Tied, and Satisfied*. This meant that for 40 days, I dominated Ian, and then we switched and Ian dominated me for the next 40 days. We worked with top kink practitioners as our coaches, and we experimented with a wide variety of kinky play.

On its own, this was an intense experience.

And shortly into Ian's 40 days of dominating me, my previous trauma began to get triggered. Playing with blindfolds and gags brought up powerful emotions and dissociated behavior.

We immediately brought in a kink-friendly and trauma-trained therapist to guide us through our experiment. We eliminated the use of blindfolds and gags. We made sure that in any role-playing scenes we engaged in, I would have full use of my voice. Ian was made aware of and kept alert for signals that could indicate I was moving into trauma response, and we continued our experiment with powerful healing taking place.

Because we had support, we navigated this treacherous territory, and I gained agency and empowerment through our experimentation.

I would not recommend that you use kink to heal. But I would say that kink, used consciously and with the guidance of skilled practitioners, may provide profound healing.

SAFETY FIRST!

Learning safe practices when using toys and gear that come along with kinky play is *mandatory*. Sensation-based play using ropes, impact, and pain-inducing implements carries serious risk of bodily harm. Even psychological kinky play that involves no physical interaction can have risks, so learn how to keep yourself safe in this kind of play as well.

Journal Quickie: Kinky Desires?

This journal exercise will help you admit all your desires to yourself. This will give you practice in communicating those desires, and maybe even help you find new turn-ons you didn't know you had.

Here are the two prompts you will use during this exercise:

Prompt 1: Share a sexual desire you have that you feel is taboo.

Prompt 2: Share something you would like others to understand about this desire.

If you are journaling, your journal entry would look like this:

Share a sexual desire you have that you feel is taboo.

I would like to have sex in a public space and have people around me as voyeurs in my pleasure.

Share something you would like others to understand about this desire.

I don't know if I really want to do this, or if it's just a hot fantasy. I'm scared of going to a sleazy swingers club—I want to do this safely and consensually.

Repeat these prompts, journaling this for at least twenty to thirty minutes. Conclude this practice by writing down any insights or knowledge you gained.

One of the Shadow sides of the Kinky realm is that people rush in without knowing what they're doing. Without some preparation and study beforehand, you may end up diving in without understanding how you and your partner(s) can keep each other safe, both physically and psychologically. It's like trying to be a pilot without any knowledge of how to do a cockpit safety check—let alone actually fly the plane! You would put yourself and all the passengers in danger.

If you want to use ropes, you need to first learn how to tell if restraints are tied too tight and which major nerves in the body could be cut off if they are.

If you want to flog or use paddles, you need to learn where on the body it's not safe to strike someone.

If you want to learn power games, you need to know which buttons not to push with your submissive partner.

The list goes on.

Learning these safety skills (and many others) from knowledgeable and ethical mentors is the best approach. See the resources at the end of this book (page 287) for information on our favorite kink experts. When you're looking for a kink practitioner, make sure to do your due diligence and check out their reputation for ethical and safe play. This is true if you're hiring any sexuality coach or practitioner, but it's especially true when you're diving into the world of kink.

The Turn-Ons of the Kinky

Kinkys are turned on by anything that is taboo for them.

It's that simple.

If it's taboo for you and it turns you on, then it's a form of kinky play . . .

And you just may be a Kinky Type.

Your turn-on might be something society has told us is taboo or something you personally think is taboo based on your lived experiences. Our culture has defined what is deemed "okay" for people of particular genders to wear, and for some strange reason, the culture says it's not okay for men to wear stockings, heels, and dresses. My client Billie was taught that wearing stockings was taboo; playing in that taboo turned him on, which is what helped him determine he was Kinky.

Here's another example. I once worked with a couple who came from a very religious background. They had had sex in the same position, on the same day of the week, and in the same exact way for the forty years they'd been together.

Why? Because anything else was taboo. Oral sex was taboo. And anal play—don't go there for sure!

They had decided that having sex in the missionary position, once a week, was what their religion deemed permissible. Eventually, this routine became so stale that they felt bored. They were in the sexual graveyard. They had become roommates, best friends who had obligatory sex once a week!

Because everything besides missionary sex was taboo for them, they both fell into the Kinky Blueprint. Having sex in new positions was so naughty and so taboo that it created intense excitement for them. Having sex multiple times a week—whoa! Now they were *really* breaking their own rules!

Adding in anal play? Well, that was so exciting and so taboo, it put them on another planet.

When we started to introduce this taboo play into their intimacy, their whole sex life was reinvigorated. No longer were they two ships passing in the night—they were now on a debauched pirate galleon, interacting with joy, fun, and playful sexuality together.

Here are some common turn-ons I see that fall within this Blueprint. By no means is this an exhaustive list—you can add more and more turn-ons depending on what is taboo for you:

» Intense sensation play (scratch, slap, sting, thud), including flogging, caning, spanking, and intense temperature play
» Role-play with power dynamics
» BDSM
» Fluid play, like being urinated on for pleasure
» Cross-dressing/gender play
» Explicit talk
» Long scenes or play sessions that involve taboo dynamics
» Psychological power games

Creating a list of all your desires is the first step in fully expressing who you are as a Kinky Type. A lot of people stop there, but I encourage you to go one step further by creating a plan to explore your turn-ons and edges.

A huge edge for me is handing over power to my lover(s) and being able to trust that they have me. Surrendering myself to someone I trust, and who has the mastery to be able to hold me erotically, is an experience I deeply desire. It took some time, coaching, and classes for me and my loves to be able to practice the power play I craved.

LET'S TALK ABOUT PAIN

While not all kink has to be painful, pain can be kinky.

Kinky interactions are multifaceted. These experiences have an impact on a variety of human mental, social, and biological processes. According to research published in the *Journal of Sexual Medicine*, pain feels good during kinky experiences because it involves the pleasure and reward systems, the stress response, pain perception, empathy-related circuits, and social interaction and bonding.

When it comes to kink, some people are sensation-based—that is, they are turned on by the intensity of the sensations. Are you turned on by the feeling of ropes, straps, or cuffs binding your body and creating constriction? This intensity of sensation and the restriction of movement creates arousal and surrender.

Embody It: Exploring Your Edgy Turn-Ons

It's time to start exploring some of the items on your list of taboo desires by learning safe and consensual ways to play with them. Take your list and circle three desires that feel like they have the least taboo and the most amount of turn-on.

Here are some examples of things you might start exploring:

» Rope Play

- Sign up for a virtual rope-tying course you can do in the comfort of your own home.
- Hire a rope expert to come do a private class for you.
- Go out to a group rope-tying class.
- Attend an event at a kink club with a group of friends and watch a rope-play scene.

» Power Play—Submissive

- Take a class on submissive personas and then embody that persona.
- Research places to find a skilled Dominant to play with.
- Find other submissives and join kink communities.

» Power Play—Dominant

- Apprentice with a kink master.
- Be submissive first so you know how it feels.
- Take classes in anything you find is a turn-on in the Dominant realm.

Take a moment now to make a list of things to play with your top three taboo turn-ons!

I have many clients who love the sensation of slapping or spanking. If you give it a try, you may be surprised to find that you too are driven wild by intensely painful play.

What do researchers have to say about why we are we turned on by pain? Let's get nerdy together!

Physical and psychological pain is a common feature of BDSM, but many people outside of the kink community find it difficult to understand why pain is pleasurable and desirable.

In 2019, a group of sexuality researchers theorized why pain might be experienced as pleasurable among those who practice BDSM. They found that the emotional, physiological, and psychological elements of pain interact to transform the experience of pain into pleasure. The experience of pain in this context can bring about expanded states of consciousness, like those that occur during mindfulness meditation.

Various factors work together to influence the experience of BDSM pain. Sexual arousal before (and/or alongside) pain acts as a pain reliever by changing the levels of dopamine and oxytocin released. So no more excuses that your headache is a reason to skip kinky sex!

When a kinky scene is set, the anticipation of pain can be what produces the sexual arousal and pleasure for the Kinky, just as the anticipation of touch is a turn-on for the Energetic.

Once pain is activated, changes occur in your dopamine, cortisol, endogenous opioids, and endogenous endocannabinoids (wow, that word turns me on) levels, influencing the psychological and physiological response to the painful sensations. In other words, you get "high" on your body's own chemicals.

This flood of nerdy words for biochemicals can send some Kinky people into "sub space," a state of euphoria, deep trance, or complete loss of oneself to time and space.

Curious about trying intense sensations now?

Let's do it.

Embody It: Sweet Spot of Pain as Pleasure

In this exercise, you can play with yourself or a willing and safe partner, or you can hire a professional sexuality educator who specializes in kink.

For this exercise, we are going to explore slapping your inner thigh. Of course, you can do this with a variety of sensations on other body parts. If you are working with a partner, discuss beforehand what sensations you want to explore. Consent is always key.

Using a cupped, relaxed hand, lightly slap your inner thigh on the same side of your body as that hand. On a scale of 1 to 10 (10 being incredibly painful and 1 being not painful at all), rate how painful you find the sensation of the slap. Now give it a pleasure rating: On a scale of 1 to 5 (5 being orgasmic and 1 being unpleasant), where would you rate this slap?

The goal of this exercise is to find the sweet spot. Keep increasing or decreasing the pain intensity if your pleasure rating is below a 3. You can also play with location. Where on your body, and with what level of impact, does the intense sensation produce a pleasure rating of 3 or higher?

This exercise is often surprising to people, and they find that with more sensation, there is often more pleasure—especially if they're wired Kinky and are more sensation-based. You can also try this exercise with impact implements such as floggers, paddles, or crops.

SENSATION-BASED OR PSYCHOLOGICAL TURN-ON

In my practice, I've noticed that some people fall within the Kinky Blueprint, but do not like impact or sensation play. Many people in our community who identify with the Kinky Blueprint find themselves loving psychological play. The difference between someone who is more sensation-based (they love the intensity of taboo sensations) and someone who is psychological-based is that the latter gets off on the game playing and power dynamics, and can sometimes orgasm or reach peak states without ever being touched. Do you have a rich fantasy world where you are the Dominant and everything is in your control? Or maybe you fantasize about being dominated and serving your lover in every way.

Ian loves the psychological aspect of this Blueprint. He likes to switch between being the one in power and the one giving power over to another.

In our dynamic, I'm often more Dominant, and he loves it when I boss him around and make him do things that are taboo for him. Ian's interest in rope play is more psychological because it makes him feel out of control, and I can do whatever I want with him.

Some people are psychologically turned on but love sensation play, too. That's Ian. As long as the psychological aspect is present and he feels the ropes binding him intensely, the turn-on goes even higher.

POSTGAME FOLLOW-UP

Playing in new territory in solo pleasure and especially in partnered pleasure can make you feel vulnerable and can set off some triggers. It's important that you communicate with your lover(s) about what works and what doesn't.

If something didn't work for you, express it from your personal experience and do not shame or blame your partner in the process, especially if they played within the rules you established before diving into the sexual experiment.

For example, instead of sharing something like, "You were so aggressive when you bossed me around. You're like that around the house and I hate it," find something authentic to say about how it felt to have your partner boss you around: "I struggled when you commanded me each time in the scene. I felt my body contract and I did not feel connected to turn-on. What I would like to try next time, so I can surrender and have more fun, is for you to gently whisper each command in my ear. Would you be willing to give that a try?"

Broken boundaries also must be addressed. If one or the other of you did not honor your container of consent, repair is needed.

Here are four postgame follow-up questions you can ask each other after any new erotic encounter.

"What worked for you about that experience?"

"What are two or three highlights that stand out for you?"

"What would you like more of if we play with this again?"

"What didn't work for you, and what would you like to try instead?"

Kinky Superpowers

As someone with a Kinky Blueprint begins to heal the Shadows and own the awesomeness of their turn-ons, they step more fully into their Superpowers. And as they own these Superpowers, they strengthen.

Here's a short list of Kinky Superpowers:

» Endless creativity

» Lots of fun gadgets and toys to explore and master

» Potential for healing and empowerment

» Surrender and deepening loving care

» Variety of orgasms, some without even being touched

» Going into expanded states of consciousness (sub space/Dom-space)

» Freedom to play with a variety of identities, role-play

Embody It: "Be the Boss" Power Game

For this exercise, you'll need a partner who is willing either to be the boss or to be submissive. As with any kink exercise, start with a consent conversation.

Remember, a yes can always become a no, but a no cannot become a yes. Ever. (For a refresher on consent conversations, see page 23.)

Agree on the amount of time you will spend playing this game. If you're new to this kind of play, make the scene short—ten to twenty minutes. Set yourself up for quick wins.

The person who is the boss will literally boss the other around, ordering them to do various activities. These can be sexual and taboo, or they can be service-oriented activities.

Here are some ideas:

» "Striptease for me."

» "Be naked around the house."

» "Self-pleasure for me."

» "Do the dishes topless."

» "Hold a sexy pose while I take your picture."

» "Let me admire you while you sit there."

» "Kiss my feet."

» "Sit at my feet while I work."

» "Don't look at me unless I instruct you to do so."

» "Go out to dinner with a remote-control vibrator in your pants, and give me the remote!"

When the allotted time is up, make sure you both praise each other for what worked well and make a note of what you would like to do more of next time.

If you are a Kinky, it's important for you to know what turns you on so that you can communicate this with your lover(s). If you aren't sure what turns you on, that process of discovery will be the start of your journey.

INFINITE CREATIVITY

One of the primary Superpowers of the Kinky is their endless creativity. They can come up with so many different and wonderful ways to explore sexuality.

I feel like I could explore within this Blueprint for the rest of my life and not come close to exhausting all the gloriously naughty possibilities. Truly, there are no limits to the variety of ways to play here.

You can come up with plenty of exciting taboos and then create whole scenes and worlds around them. I've seen kink performances that went on for hours. They were edgy, erotic, smoldering, humorous, and profound.

I highly encourage you to go watch some kink performances yourself to experience a whole new realm of creative sexual play. There are often kink events at clubs in major cities that show everything from flogging and rope play to pet play (the pony shows are amazing) and fire play.

TOUCHLESS ORGASMS, TOO

Like Energetics, Kinkys can have orgasms without sexual stimulation. Due to the psychological aspect of this Blueprint, orgasm and high pleasure can come from the stimulation of the mind. I have been witness to some incredible orgasms coming from psychological play and intense sensation play that never touched the genitals. I once saw a whipping demonstration where, as the whip got closer and closer to the woman's body, she became more and more aroused. With her legs spread, and after a number of loud snaps of the whip just inches from her vulva, she began to orgasm. That's the power of Kinky anticipation.

So Your Lover Is a Kinky . . .

If you're just now discovering your lover is a Kinky, it can be a little over-whelming. Your mind might make up all kinds of stories about what this means. Do your best not to let your mind run away with all kinds of fears that may not even be real concerns. And if they *are* real, it's important not to judge or shame your Kinky partner. Just because your lover has a specific desire or fetish does not require you to be the one to fulfill their cravings.

Be as accepting as you can, and get support for yourself and your part-ner. If it all feels like it's too much for you, hire a coach who specializes in kink. (See the resources section on page 287 to find out how to locate an expert to work with.)

STEP ONE: ACCEPTANCE AND SAFETY

The first step is to create a safe space for your lover to express themselves and to share what really turns them on. Really ask yourself if you can provide that safe space for your partner to share without judgment or shame.

What many Kinky people fear most is that they will be shamed, judged, abandoned, or harmed for their desires. The most important thing you can do is to be as accepting as you can, and even to cheer them on as they explore their newfound sexual expression. Seek to understand them, and try not to make it about you. To start, make it clear that you want to explore kink collaboratively with your partner, and if need be, that they take the lead in this exploration.

And remember, acts that are not consensual are not kink. These acts are often abusive behavior. If you find yourself in this circumstance, stopping this behavior and getting support is imperative.

STEP TWO: SKILLS

In the arena of kink, I highly recommend that you learn as much as you can about the things that turn your partner on. If they love ropes, go take a class on various rope ties. If they love the psychological aspect, go take classes on submission and Dominance. If they love alien role-play games, go shopping for some fun costumes.

Showing that you are willing to learn and play with them goes a very long way to creating safety and feeding a Kinky Blueprint.

Show them you are willing to take the time to learn about them and to learn the skills to turn them on. Then do it!

One of the essential learnings for anyone with a Kinky partner is how to be sensitive to the shame a Kinky can harbor. Come to your lover with an air of curiosity, never judgment. Curiosity always breeds intimacy and connection; judgment shuts it down in an instant.

STEP THREE: FREEDOM

It took a lot of work for me to be able to come to my lovers who were Kinky. I had to unravel all the myths and misunderstandings I was harboring. It took years of training to be able to bring any level of mastery to them. And I had to give them the freedom to explore erotically what I couldn't provide. I'm not saying that you must do anything you don't want to do, but in myself, I have found a love that allows others to be fully expressed in who they are without me restricting them.

It's advanced work, with any Erotic Blueprint Type, to get to that place where you love and accept your lover so deeply that you realize you do not own them or their body. You can give them the freedom to explore all their desires. And then you both become free to express yourselves erotically, without judgment, shame, or restriction.

Journal Quickie: Rating Your Taboos

Make a list of all your taboo desires (you can use the list you made during the Journal Quickie on page 161). Next, on a scale of 1 to 10 (10 being the most taboo and 1 being the least), rate each desire on how taboo it feels for you and mark this number next to the item on your list.

Now note if you feel shame, turn-on, or both for each of these desires.

Where to Begin If You Are Kinky

If you find yourself relating to this Blueprint and you've discovered that you are indeed Kinky, congratulations!

If you were disturbed to discover you have Kinky inclinations, or you're wishing you weren't turned on by the taboo, then it's time to do a little work on excavating and healing shame. The work for you is twofold: The first part is looking at the shame and the parts of you that feel shame for your desires. The second part is laying out and owning all your desires.

We aren't trying to get rid of the taboo feeling—the taboo is where the turn-on is. What we're trying to do is to look at the shame you're harboring about the taboo turn-on. When you look at the desire, do you feel the juice and the aliveness of the taboo, or do you feel shame?

Shame is destructive. You beat yourself up with it. You are not in acceptance of who you are and what turns you on. Taboo feels good. Taboo says, "Ooooooh, isn't that juicy? Isn't that full of life force? I love that naughty, naughty thing, even though I feel like I shouldn't! I'm amazing!"

It's important to distinguish and separate out the exciting taboo from the shame. It's important that you feel the difference in the mind chatter.

All right, my naughty kitty cats, on that note, it's time to move into a world where you love it all, you want it all, and you want it all the time.

If you've found turn-on in all the Blueprints we've explored so far, well, the next chapter is definitely for you. And because I know you want more and more and more, I'm going to give it to you!

CHAPTER ELEVEN

the shapeshifter

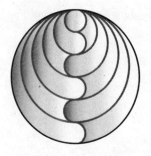

I want it all. I want it now.

—QUEEN

You Might Be a Shapeshifter Blueprint If . . .

» You relate to all the desires, wants, and needs of the other four Blueprint Types.

» You have a voracious appetite for and are turned on by everything erotic. You want it all, you want more of it, and you want it all the time.

» You can ride endless waves of pleasure and sustain heightened arousal for hours upon hours.

» During a lovemaking session, your lover is spent when you feel like you've barely just begun.

» You are highly erotically sophisticated and have played with, or want to play with, every form of erotic expression.

» You are a versatile, confident lover, able to satisfy your partner no matter what Blueprint Type they are.

» You find yourself shapeshifting to meet your lover's wants and desires, but your needs are never fully met. You feel unseen and unmet in the bedroom, and you're left starving for sexual fulfillment.

» People have repeatedly said things to you like "You're too much" or "You're too complicated."

Imagine a world where every erotic treat, a buffet of orgasmic delights, is there for your taking. Every flavor awaits your tongue. Every sensation begs to dance on your skin.

And you get to have it all at once, and you get to have it all, all the time! Welcome to the realm of the Shapeshifter.

The Shapeshifter Shadow

"It's like I'm a bottomless pit!" Randi exclaimed. "I can have one orgasm, and then I want another. Honestly, after an hour my lovers complain they are tired. Where's the off button?"

I could see Randi squirming in embarrassment. Her cheeks flushed red as she so effusively revealed this big challenge in her sex life.

Randi had recently found out that she is a Shapeshifter, and she was struggling with understanding the positive Superpowers of this Blueprint. She was clearly stuck in the Shadow side and hadn't yet seen the light of possibility that this Blueprint provided.

"Dating has become harder now that I know I'm a Shapeshifter. I can't have five people all go home with me every night just to make sure I'm fed! Not to mention, I must teach them all this complexity. And I don't feel satisfied unless I have it all," Randi continued, and the distress in her body heightened.

"I could go back to just pleasing everyone else. I can shift into what they want. It wasn't that bad. It seemed a whole lot easier than trying to get my needs met." She was near tears now, her voice cracking and becoming high-pitched.

Is a Shapeshifter too much?

So often I hear from a Shapeshifter's lovers that their sexual cravings are just overwhelming. And Shapeshifters judge themselves as being too much, oftentimes because somewhere early in their sexual lifetime they were told this.

Along with the too-muchness, Shapeshifters are often told—and come to believe—that they're too complex. While it may seem that Shapeshifters are complex, this is not the truth—they're just the most erotically intelligent and sophisticated of all the Blueprints. I'll touch on that more when we talk about their scrumptious Superpowers.

STARVATION, SATIATION, AND SHIFTING TO PLEASE

Often, because Shapeshifters are so fabulous, the biggest Shadow they deal with is that they tend to shift into whatever their lover's Blueprint is.

Randi believed that she was too much and too complex, so wouldn't it be better for her to just do what Shapeshifters do best and shift herself to meet her lover's needs?

It can be fulfilling to have the Superpower of being the ultimate lover . . .

But it comes with a cost.

Randi knew deep down that she'd spent most of her sexual life thus far pleasing others and had always left sexual encounters feeling only somewhat satisfied. Her last partner was a Sexual, and she had felt like she was always having intercourse and quickies, and while the sex was good, it didn't scratch the itch. Her partner was unwilling to meet her desire for variety or to try anything outside of the Sexual Blueprint.

After their breakup, she started dating and finding pleasure in having many lovers. However, unaware she was a Shapeshifter, and still caught in the Shadow side of her Blueprint, she kept switching to meet their needs. She was becoming great at pleasing others, but felt continually unsatisfied herself.

Now that she was aware of her Blueprint Type, she was starting to do things differently, but she wanted more, and more, and more . . .

Pleasure First: Scintillating Shapeshifter Sensations

Let's explore a wide variety of sensations all over your body! You can use your hands and sensation play items. Take up to five minutes to explore each different type of touch.

Begin by hovering your hands over your body, in just the way that an Energetic would love. Next, let your fingertips lightly dance over your skin. Go slowly, breathe, and simply notice how this feels. Now move into Sensual contouring touch on your skin or use your favorite sensation toys.

Keep breathing, because there's more.

Next, begin to explore your genitals. What would turn you on the most and bring you the most pleasure? Your favorite vibrator? Long, slow strokes? Penetration?

Keep breathing—there's more.

Deny yourself a progression to orgasm. Slap your inner thighs, scratch your chest, or try a few sensation items.

And finally, experiment with putting it all together.

Can you ride that vibrator while you lightly dance on your skin with one hand and use the other to sensually caress, then cap it off with a slap of surprise? Can you touch your genitals with one hand while the other pulls your hair? Oh, the possibilities are endless!!!

I know it seems harder than rubbing your tummy and patting your head at the same time, but for a Shapeshifter, this is a normal Tuesday!

For this Pleasure First, you are encouraged to climax or orgasm.

Notice the effects of this practice on your body. Did it overwhelm you? Do you feel like you could go for more?

Because Shapeshifters are so multifaceted, have a huge appetite for variety, are often at a high level of erotic mastery, and can take so much pleasure, they are often left feeling unsatiated.

Feeling satiation is an important practice for anyone who can take more and more, and who wants a level of skillful mastery from their lovers that surpasses their wildest dreams.

Randi started to get very critical of her past lover and the lovers she was currently dating. "I just feel like I'm light-years ahead of everyone sexually. Why can't I find someone who can please all of me?" she complained. "Especially the Sexuals—I mean, there's a time and a place for that, but going right for my genitals without anything else all the time? It's just boring!" She rolled her eyes as she slammed the other Blueprints. I could see that so much of her judgment was simply coming from her past experiences and the pain of pleasure starvation.

I've seen Shapeshifters like Randi who, even after multiple lovers and having many hands all over their bodies for hours, are still desirous of more pleasure. They have such a huge capacity, which is wonderful, but at the same time can be hard for lovers of Shapeshifters who don't have that same sex drive. Their lovers also may not have the mastery that such fine-tuned instruments as Shapeshifters desire (especially Energetic Shapeshifters).

I believe that part of the reason Shapeshifters want more and more is that they've spent so much of their sexual lifetime in a space of erotic starvation. And there's nothing wrong with wanting more—it's when that craving becomes a distressing hunt that problems arise.

A Shapeshifter can start to chase big ecstatic peak experiences, always looking for the next high and never integrating or having the ability to just be.

After Randi discovered more about the Shadows specific to the Shapeshifter Blueprint, we started to look at the Shadow sides of all the other Blueprints.

I wanted to see if perhaps she was what I call a Shadow Shapeshifter.

THE SHADOW SHAPESHIFTER

The Shadow Shapeshifter is a Shapeshifter who has all the Shadows of every Blueprint Type, but very few, or none, of their Superpowers.

Can you imagine the frustration and pain of living with all the Shadows of the four other Blueprint Types? It can be a long and difficult journey for someone who has developed as a Shadow Shapeshifter, but it's not a hopeless one. Once the Shadows are given voice and a space to be safe, they can be transformed and blossom into full Superpowers.

Randi's Shadows were mostly specific to the Shapeshifter, but she had built up some Energetic Shadows as well. She was judgmental of other Blueprints, especially the Sexual, and she had a hard time stating what she needed.

Shapeshifters are often told they are too much, which can shut them down, or told they are too complex or complicated, when the truth is that they are just erotically sophisticated. Shapeshifters are constantly shifting to please their lovers, which often leaves them starving in their own sexuality. They may feel dissatisfied with the quantity and quality of the sex they are getting and may have a hard time feeling satiation. They also have most of the Shadows of all the other Blueprints, but very few of their Superpowers and turn-ons.

If you deeply relate to these Shadows, you may be interested in how to heal or integrate them. In chapter fifteen, I'll touch on healing the Shadow side of your Blueprints. In the meantime, I want to leave you with the way in which Randi began to work with the Shadows.

After doing the Bringing the Light to the Shadows exercise with each of the Shadows, Randi was able to cultivate new beliefs and thoughts that started to free her from the constraints she was putting on herself. New ideas began to emerge, and she was more able to step into her Superpowers and turn-ons without restriction.

Shapeshifter Turn-Ons

Oh, the marvelous, wonderful, delicious, cosmic, sexual, kinky places you can go!

Shapeshifters, when fully cultivated, are turned on by absolutely everything.

They can be turned on by all things cosmic and otherworldly like the Energetic. They can find utter delight in the delicious full-body pleasure of the Sensual. Sexual sex can bring them to intense climax. And they find pleasure in the Kinky's huge variety of turn-ons.

There are turn-ons specific to the Shapeshifter themselves, too:

» Feeling attunement and sexual mastery from a lover
» Mixing and blending the Blueprints together
» Having lots of space and time for erotic play
» Being in a space where there's a lot of variety and plenty of options for sexual play
» Getting the opportunity to shapeshift and show off their Superpowers and skills in both giving and receiving
» Being acknowledged as erotically intelligent instead of being told they are complex and complicated
» Inviting them into more pleasure and challenging them on how much pleasure they can take
» Giving them the experience of many hands on their body or lovers to play with (if they are in an open relationship or practicing nonmonogamy)
» Self-pleasure sessions that include a journey through all the Erotic Blueprints

Journal Quickie:
Bringing Light to the Shadows

Choose any Shapeshifter Shadow that you are working with.
Write a short statement at the top of a page in your journal
about the problem with that Shadow. For example: *I never feel
satisfied when it comes to sex.*

. Then write four brief sentences about what you wrote at the
top of the page that express how you feel about this statement.
For example:

1. I'm really angry that people are so uneducated about sex.
2. I fear I'm always going to be this way.
3. I wish I didn't demand so much from my lovers.
4. Why can't I just be one thing instead of so complicated?

Next, reread each sentence and notice what images come up in
your mind, what thoughts arise about that sentence, what emotions
you are feeling, and what body sensations occur as you read.

Now write three brief sentences to articulate how you feel
about what you originally wrote at the top of the page. How do
you feel about that problem now?

For example:

1. I wish I had a lover who could meet all my needs.
2. What would it take to feel really satisfied?
3. Maybe I'm making this a bigger issue than it really is.

Do the same method of rereading each sentence and feeling
the image, thought, emotion, and bodily sensation as you
reread them.

Now write two brief sentences about how you feel and reread them.

Now write one brief sentence.

If that last sentence doesn't feel positive and good, then keep going. You want to get to at least three positive sentences in a row.

Write two sentences and reread.

Write three sentences and reread.

Write four sentences and reread.

Then reverse the process and go back down to one. Keep going until you have at least three sentences that feel positive and good.

In truth, there is no limit to what can arouse a Shapeshifter!

At one of our advanced-level live events, we have an entire Shapeshifter day, where people get the opportunity to have an experience of pleasure that includes all the Erotic Blueprints stacked together.

We invite participants to bring all their favorite pleasure items and to come with lots of creative ideas about how to be fed. There is an opportunity for a huge variety of pleasure and a whole lot of it. Participants work in groups of four, and the experience starts with a deep consent conversation and a voicing of desires the night before. I am always impressed by what Shapeshifters come up with! This experience can get wild and fun and so free. Many participants report to us that it was a life-changing experience.

And can you guess what the number one complaint at the end of a six-handed, three-hour Shapeshifter experience is?

There wasn't enough time!

Once a Shapeshifter has moved from the Shadows, their turn-ons truly become unlimited. Randi was so pleased when it seemed like overnight, she was turned on by anything and everything.

"It's like it doesn't matter anymore what I'm playing with. It's all become a turn-on for me! I'm so happy! And so grateful!" She beamed brightly at me. "I still want more, but it's different. Now it feels like I only want more because it's all so delightful and creative. The possibilities for my sexuality seem endless," she exclaimed.

It's true—the possibilities are endless for Shapeshifters. But I also believe that they're endless for all of us, no matter what Blueprint we most identify with.

In time, thanks to clients like Randi, I came to believe that deep down, we are all Shapeshifters.

Discovering our Primary Erotic Blueprint is incredibly empowering and shows us where we have the easiest, most resourced access to arousal and sexual satisfaction. Identifying only with this Primary Blueprint, however, shows us where we are limited. If you only play with the pleasures of your Primary Blueprint, you're missing out on most of the orgasmic buffet laid out before you.

Truly we are all full-spectrum erotic beings who have a huge capacity for pleasure, play, and deep personal awakening. The opportunity is there for all of us to explore and expand into all that is erotically possible.

As Randi stepped more and more into letting go of limiting Shadows and became deeply fed in her core Shapeshifter turn-ons, her ability to tap into her fullness grew and grew. She began seeing the malleability of her identity, and the less fixed she became in one identity, the more she stepped into who she really is.

She began to experience the multitudes of her true self. And the more she stepped into that truth, the more everything became possible for her.

Shapeshifter Superpowers

Shapeshifters, when fully developed into their Superpowers, amaze us all!

They can dance in the mystical realms of the Energetic. They can luxuriate in the full-body sensuality of the Sensual. They can dive right into the pleasures of orgasmic satiation of the Sexual. They can find mastery in the art of the taboo that the Kinky so loves. And on top of that, they have all their own Shapeshifter Superpowers, which, even after almost thirty years of practice, still surprise me.

Here are some Shapeshifter Superpowers we can all get excited about:

» Fully developing all the Superpowers of all the Blueprints
» Expanding beyond fixed identities and having true freedom to be anything you choose to be
» Unlimited turn-ons, unlimited variety of play, unlimited unlimitedness
» Becoming a true master of sexuality and pleasure
» Learning how to generate your own peak experiences and settling more deeply into peak existence—"being" instead of "doing" or "receiving"
» Having realizations and experiences that show you how sex is a tool for awakening to your true self

Does all this sound exciting to you?

One of my moments with Randi became my favorite moment of working with any client. She came to me with tears of joy streaming down her face as she laughed. It's the laugh I love so much—there's nothing like that laugh, and words wouldn't do it justice.

She looked me right in the eyes.

"Fuck!" she exclaimed. "Oh, fuck!" She threw her hands in the air. "Really?" She laughed again. I knew this truth she had just glimpsed because I have felt this truth myself.

"All of that, everything, led here, now! Fuck!"

I smiled at her and nodded.

"I'm me. This is. I'm here. Hi!" She laughed again. And we just laughed and cried together. No more words were needed.

She had directly experienced the truth of who and what she is. She had felt it to her core. And she was transformed.

Some of you will read this and think that this experience is something to attain, some state you can get to, some peak experience you will begin to chase until you can catch it.

But the moment you chase it, it will elude you. Because chasing takes you away from the pleasure of the present-moment experience.

In my deepest truth, I believe that when sex is truly honored for what it is meant to be, practiced at its grandest level, this is what happens.

We have the capacity to realize who and what we are, and for a moment, all the seeking, chasing, and trying to be something, to be enough, stops.

We stop running away or toward something, and we relax into the recognition of this unified moment. And here we are.

Perhaps this happens because by the time we fully develop into being Shapeshifters, we've exhausted all the routes of endless seeking.

True satiation arises.

When we give up chasing or running, something amazing can happen. We can just be. We can just be who we truly are, and we realize that we are the ones who generate our own pleasure. We are pleasure itself. We are joy itself. We are love itself.

We no longer need to chase some sexual ideal to attain anything. We are inherently worthy. We are freedom itself. We are love. Sex becomes creative play, and is no longer a place where we go to fulfill something or get away from something. There is nothing else in this world like this feeling.

So Your Lover Is a Shapeshifter . . .

If you're not a Shapeshifter yourself, having a partner who is a Shapeshifter may feel foreign and overwhelming.

Not to worry! You can learn to feed your Shapeshifter partner by being willing to learn to master your own Primary and Secondary Erotic Blueprints.

I'm big on creating easy wins for yourself. Can you take classes to deepen your knowledge and skills on how to give pleasure in that Blueprint? Once you feel like you've gained some mastery with your Primary Blueprint, move to your Secondary Blueprint. Keep studying and exploring until you have skills in all the Blueprints.

Being willing to learn, practice, and play is a key to lifelong sexual satisfaction. Understanding that learning about sex is a lifelong adventure will help you stay open to mastery.

One of the best gifts you can give your Shapeshifter partner is to encourage their expansiveness and acknowledge their erotic intelligence.

Love who they are. Love the variety and multitude of turn-ons they bring. Understand that they love when you show interest in learning how to improve your sex skills and do your best to not take it personally when they want more or are feeling dissatisfied. The more sex skills you learn and the more you execute what you learn, the more you will feed them.

Get creative, use a lot of variety, and stay curious about who they are and what they love. Sometimes you must really put your ego aside when it comes to feeding a Shapeshifter (or any Blueprint that you don't understand). The Shapeshifter can easily get triggered and feel hopeless if you get defensive or try to claim that you know everything already.

Feeding your Shapeshifter lover takes some erotic expansion on your part. If you are willing to do the work and play necessary, and they can learn to trust you on your journey, you'll find that in the end, you just might become a Shapeshifter along with them!

That's the biggest benefit: they will challenge you into your own expansion. That expansion is the greatest gift you can give them, and it will be a gift to you as well.

Where to Begin If You're a Shapeshifter

I have a couple of suggestions to help you. But you might want to start with some deep breaths. Shapeshifters can sometimes overwhelm themselves!

STEP ONE: ACCEPTANCE

Start in a place of deep acceptance. You are big. You are sophisticated erotically. You are a symphony orchestra with fine instruments just waiting for the right virtuoso to come and play you!

It's time for you to accept just how magnificent you are. And, from that place, to be compassionate toward yourself and show compassion for your lovers. After all, no one taught them how to play a symphony orchestra, and all at once!

STEP TWO: GET FED

I know you've been patient. I know you may be starving right now, but trust me when I say that once you know who you are, you can begin the journey of getting your needs truly met.

Begin by making a list of ways that you would like to play.

What feels truly fulfilling to you? What are things you would like to experience? Make a sexual bucket list and begin pursuing each experience, marking them off one by one by one.

STEP THREE: HEAL YOUR SHADOWS

If you are caught deeply in the Shadow of this Blueprint, you may want to do some clearing and healing of those Shadow parts so you can fully step into freely exploring all the possibilities on your bucket list. (I'll go more deeply into healing the Shadows in chapter fifteen.)

STEP FOUR: PRACTICE SATIATION

What is the experience of being completely satiated? How does deep satisfaction feel? Can you generate that experience from within? Introspection is a great place for a Shapeshifter to begin!

Congratulations! We have now looked at and experienced each of the five Erotic Blueprints. We've had a bit of a mental journey so far, and now it's time to go deeper into your body. In the next chapter, I'm going to give you guidelines on how to uncover anyone's Blueprint through hands-on practices that allow the body to speak its truth.

CHAPTER TWELVE

determining erotic blueprints

I believe that the body never lies. It will tell you what it feels—if you listen.

Now, sometimes your body may be at odds with your mind. But when you manage to get them both on the same page, some magical things can happen. As a somatic (meaning "body-based") sexologist, I know just how glorious and amazing our bodies are. If we didn't have bodies to feel sensations, sex would be so bland, so blah!

Your body has a lot to tell you, and a lot of experiences to bring you. And we've reached the time for you to deepen your relationship with your body so that you can take the next step on your journey of erotic awakening.

Pleasure First: Body Talk

This exercise is an opportunity to surrender.

Leave at least twenty minutes for this exercise.

Lie down comfortably on your back.

Put your hands anywhere on your body where they are intuitively drawn. Notice the rise and fall of your breath and begin to drop into your body with your awareness.

Now, I want you to say hello to your body as if you were greeting a wise guide who has been waiting for you to realize that they are there. Just listen for a response. The response from your body may come in words, images, bodily sensations, or even an emotional uprising. Don't worry if you don't experience anything right away. Be patient, sit with your body, and wait for its response.

Keep listening.

As things arise, do not run from those experiences. Get curious about them. You can even ask your body questions like "What would you like to communicate to me?" Or "What would bring you pleasure right now?"

After the twenty minutes are complete, say goodbye to your body for now and let it know that you will return.

Take some time to write in your journal about what was pleasurable and what you discovered.

Evolving research indicates that practicing mindfulness-based exercises like this may be very effective in restoring connectivity to the brain's networks. This will allow a person's brain impacted by stress to turn off the overactivity or avoid a shutdown.

So far in this book, we've been exploring the Blueprints from the perspective of your mind, your intellect, and what you think might (or might not) bring you pleasure. What Erotic Blueprint Type do you *think* you are?

In this chapter, I'm going to give you some embodied exercises to help you *feel* which type you may be. These exercises build on each other and go from simple to more complex. Playing in the body will give you another approach on this adventure. And what you discover may surprise you, because it isn't about what you think. If you haven't already, now may be the time to take the In-Depth Erotic Blueprint Quiz (see page 287 for more information).

Mapping Your Erotic Body

"*Ooohhhh, uuuhhh.*" A deep, guttural moan escaped her lips.

Her partner had a huge smile on his face as he held her wrists down. Her eyes started rolling back in her head. "*Uhhhhh*" was all she could muster. She was in so much pleasure. He slapped her inner thigh and her back arched, her head fell back, her mouth opened, her breathing became labored.

Just two hours before, Alison had told me she had no Kinky in her Blueprint. She was purely Sensual.

We had arranged the room to appease her Sensual Shadow, we had given her lots of Sensual touch, but nothing lit her body up like putting on leather boots and then being spanked by her partner and held down.

No Kinky in her Blueprint, huh?

It wasn't the first time I'd seen this.

"On a scale of one to five, how pleasurable is that?" I asked her as she writhed around on the massage table. Her partner had just put his hands around her neck.

"Five! *Uuuhhhhhh*," she moaned.

Just moments before this admission that choking turned her on, she'd also exclaimed during the session that slaps were a five and that holding her down was a five. Turns out she was a lot more Kinky than her mind had let on.

And that's the beauty of seeing what the body has to say.

"I can't believe that I'm Kinky," she said when she could put words together again and we were integrating her experience. "I mean, I guess it makes sense that I would discredit it." She looked at her husband. "After all, it seems it's so taboo for us, as I am a Christian."

She giggled, her face blushing. "But that was so awesome to discover after twenty-five years of being married." She leaned into her husband; a sly grin emerged on her lips. "I have to get some of these boots!"

He just smiled from ear to ear.

Many of the people I work with find themselves surprised when their body shows them that unexpected things turn them on. Either they had never tried those things before, so it's a first, or they had never had a skilled instructor there to guide them through a masterful experience of that pleasure possibility.

I first learned how to create an Erotic Map through something called body mapping, which was taught to me by Joseph Kramer, the creator of Sexological Bodywork. When you are body mapping, you are literally creating a pleasure map of the entire body.

I later learned, when studying kink, how to do comparative touch using an A/B game of mapping. With the A/B game, you compare two different kinds of touches. It's like when you go to the eye doctor and they have you choose which of two different lenses helps you see better. Do you see better with A or with B? In this case, we're determining which touch, A or B, is more pleasurable. My favorite discovery session to teach clients is a three-hour embodied experience where we use both body mapping and the A/B game to help them understand, from a somatic point of view, more of what turns them on.

Doing this with couples is extremely eye-opening and usually transforms their sexual lives together. If you don't have a partner to play with, you can try it out on your own. In the following exercises, I'm going to give you tools to map your body on your own or with your partner.

A/B GAME FOR DETERMINING YOUR BLUEPRINT

For this game, you can play solo or with a partner. If playing with a partner, make sure you have a solid consent conversation before you begin (see chapter two), especially if you've invited a friend or new lover to come play with you; do this even if you've been in the relationship for decades.

Don't let being partnerless hold you back from playing; you can always do this as a solo game, or you can find people you trust to explore with you and set clear boundaries for your game—together. We've heard many stories of people having "Blueprint determining" parties, where guests play the A/B game with friends over the course of an evening.

Make sure that you reserve uninterrupted time and space for this exercise, ideally sixty to ninety minutes at minimum for each person receiving.

In this game, as the receiver, you will be presented with two different sensations, from which you'll choose the one that brings you more pleasure.

Here's a list of items to gather to make this successful:

» Sensation play items for each Erotic Blueprint:
- Energetic: crystals, light feathers, chime
- Sensual: fur mitts, massage oil, a spoon
- Sexual: vibrator, dildo, butt toy
- Kinky: fork, nipple clamps, paddle
- Shapeshifter: any combination of the above together

» A massage table (if you don't have one, have towels or a moisture-proof blanket like a Liberator Fascinator throw to put on your bed)
» A playlist that you find sensually pleasing
» Your hands
» Your journal

IF PRACTICING SOLO, begin by giving yourself contrasting touches using tools for each Blueprint, beginning with these five A/B pairs.

Here are some other examples:

» A: Light touch with a fur mitt on your shoulder—*Energetic*
» B: Scratching with a fork down your arm—*Kinky*

» A: Slapping your inner thigh—*Kinky*
» B: Energetically hovering over your low abdomen—*Energetic*

» A: Light fingertip touch on your arms—*Energetic*
» B: Vibrator on your pubic bone—*Sexual*

» A: Fur on your genitals with vibrator on top—*Shapeshifter*
» B: Massaging your feet—*Sensual*

» A: Nipple clamps on your nipples—*Kinky*
» B: Touching your genitals—*Sexual*

As a general rule, give yourself a few minutes with each sensation. Make note of which sensation you find more pleasurable from each pair.

After you've gone through your body with a variety of touches and sensation items and compared them to each other, take some time to notice how you feel. Take a moment to journal what you've discovered from the practice.

IF PLAYING WITH A PARTNER, begin by deciding who will be the giver and who will be the receiver.

The giver will start to give contrasting touches in each Blueprint to the receiver. For example, if you give Sensual touch with fur as A, contrast it with some Kinky touch like scratching with a fork for B.

Here are some other examples:

» A: Hover your hands high above your partner and intend to send energy to them—*Energetic*
» B: Feed your partner a strawberry while lightly stroking your fingertips between their breasts—*Shapeshifter*

» A: Massage your lover's breasts—*Sensual*
» B: Pull your lover's pubic hair—*Kinky*

» A: Give your partner a pinch on their inner thigh—*Kinky*
» B: Run your fingertips over your partner's thigh—*Energetic*

» A: Kiss your lover gently—*Sensual*
» B: Rub your lover's clitoris with your fingertip (use lube)—*Sexual*

If you are the giver, make it a point to try these contrasting touches and sensations on all parts of your partner's body. Try parts of the body you wouldn't normally explore during sex, like an elbow or a pinkie finger. Make note of which sensations your partner is liking the most and the areas of the body where those sensations are highly pleasurable for them.

Give your partner a few minutes with each sensation, and don't rush the process. Focus on providing a variety of sensations, and be open to returning to certain tools if your partner asks you to.

If your lover frequently finds both sensations equally pleasurable, they are most likely a Shapeshifter. Try comparing one Blueprint (such as Energetic) to a combination of Blueprints (such as Kinky and Sensual paired together at the same time) to see what is more pleasurable.

After you've each taken a turn as the giver and the receiver, take some time to breathe together in stillness and silence. Notice how you both feel after the practice. Take a moment to talk about or journal what you've discovered, but make sure you give your lover time and space before overwhelming them with a discussion.

You may be wondering what this A/B exercise really reveals, and why it's so important to try. Well, in my years working with clients, I've seen that playing these games shows them things about their bodies they never knew. And for the first time, they are free of thought and deeply embodied.

We are all different. No two sessions are alike—one part of a person's body may light up to a specific style of touch, while another part of their body flinches or retreats from the same touch. For example, your neck may erupt in arousal with Energetic touch, but Energetic touch on your belly may feel like bugs crawling on your skin.

To build on the A/B game, let's dive into another discovery session: body mapping!

SOLO BODY-MAPPING JOURNEY

For this journey, you will need the following:

» Uninterrupted and sensuous space to practice in

» Your hands

» Sensation play items

» Ideas for different kinds of touch in each Blueprint

» Knowledge of the rating scale (explained on the following page)

» A timer

» Your journal

Please leave sixty to ninety minutes for this journey.

During this body-mapping journey, you will be going through your body with various touches and sensations. You will rate each touch/sensation on a scale of 1 to 5.

1 = Do not like this

2 = Meh, nothing special

3 = That feels good

4 = Wow, that's really pleasurable

5 = That's orgasmic!

Begin by undressing as much as you are comfortable. Naked is wonderful, if you're comfortable with it, because you can explore everywhere on your body with all the Blueprints. I instruct most of my clients to begin with Energetic touch because it provides a level of safety for most bodies.

Let's begin.

Start hovering your hands above a part of your body. How does this feel? Rate your pleasure on the scale of 1 to 5.

If it's not too disruptive, make a note in your journal as to what touches are a 3 or above—especially if they surprise you. Anything that's a 3 or above is in your turn-on zone, and remember, you are making a map for your own self-touch and self-pleasure.

Here are some ideas for touch in each Blueprint to help you explore more fully:

» Energetic:
- Hovering touch, but not actually touching—play with various distances from your body
- Light fingertip touch in circles over your joints
- Light fingertip touch on erogenous zones
- Touching the hairs on your body with a hovering touch
- Using a crystal on or above your skin

» Sensual:
- Soft-, fuzzy-, and furry-textured sensation items on your skin
- Contouring touch
- Long massage strokes with warm oil
- Feeding yourself delicious fruits or chocolate
- Stroking your hair over your own skin (if it's long enough to do so)

» Sexual:
- Touching your genitals
- Using a vibrator
- Penetration with fingers, insertable, or penis
- Self-stimulation
- Playing with your nipples
- Anal exploration

» Kinky:
- Scratching your skin
- Slapping your inner thighs
- Squeezing your arms or legs
- Playing with impact toys
- Exploring anything that feels taboo

» Shapeshifter:
- Blending any of the above with two, three, or more sensations simultaneously
- Using one hand to stimulate your genitals while the other does light Energetic touch
- Using toys to add sensations while your hands perform other touches that contrast the sensations of the toys

Throughout the journey, explore different areas of your body.

Start with your feet and work your way up to your head, exploring with each Blueprint as you go. You may find areas on your body that you never knew could provide pleasure. Sex is a whole-body experience.

At the end of your journey, take some time to notice the sensations in your body and to be with those sensations. What can you take away from this practice about being present with your body and the sensations you've explored?

You may want to take a moment to also journal about anything that surprised you. If you didn't jot down which sensations you rated over a 3 during the experience, you may want to note those now. When you take note of what works for your body, you become more aware of your pleasure and can better communicate it to your partner. That will help them bring you the satisfaction that you crave.

PARTNERED BODY-MAPPING IMMERSION

For this journey, you will need the following:

  » A willing partner to play with you
  » Uninterrupted and sensuous space to practice in
  » Sensation play items
  » Ideas for different kinds of touch in each Blueprint
  » Knowledge of the rating scale (explained on the following page)
  » A timer
  » Your journal

Please leave ninety minutes to two hours for this journey.

During this body-mapping journey, your partner will explore your body with various touches and sensations.

After they give you each sensation, they will ask you: "On a scale of one to five, how pleasurable is this?" You will rate each touch or sensation according to this scale.

1 = Do not like this

2 = Meh, nothing special

3 = That feels good

4 = Wow, that's really pleasurable

5 = That's orgasmic!

Begin with a consent conversation with your partner (see page 23), even if they have been your lover for a long time. Take a moment to express your gratitude to each other, which goes a long way in creating the loving and generous relationship that you desire.

Establish who will be the giver and who will be the receiver.

Start by undressing as much as you are comfortable. Naked is wonderful, if you're comfortable with it, because you and your partner can explore everywhere on your body with all the Blueprints.

As you go through the practice, it's important to remember that all you're doing is gathering information—there is no right or wrong. It's simply what your body likes in that moment. So be sure to embrace curiosity and openness and let go of criticism and judgment.

In this exercise, you will try the same type of touch, such as circling with light fingers or scratching gently with a fork, on different parts of the body. Remember to pay attention to parts of the body you wouldn't normally touch during sex. This is the point of body mapping.

I instruct most of my clients to begin with Energetic touch because it provides a level of safety for most bodies.

Ask for feedback as you explore each zone of the body.

Once the whole back or front side of the body is complete in one Blueprint, move to mapping the next Blueprint.

What do you notice as a result of this practice of being really present with your body and the sensations you've explored?

You may want to take a moment to journal about how this experience was for you and anything that surprised you. If you didn't do so already, you may want to write down any touches that you gave a score of 3 or more, because these are in your turn-on zone.

Olivia's Body-Mapping Miracle

When Olivia and her husband came to me, they were on the verge of divorce. They loved each other a lot but couldn't figure out the "sex part" of their relationship. Five years prior to coming to see me, Olivia had suffered a medical trauma during sex, and had almost died. Consequently, she was afraid to be in her body. To make matters worse, during their entire twenty-year marriage, she had found her husband's touch off-putting and not at all the way she wanted to be touched. But she didn't know how to communicate that to him without hurting his feelings. He'd completely lost his confidence and was resistant to trying things that so far hadn't worked in his favor. He felt utterly defeated, and felt responsible for the widening chasm between them.

After three hours of mapping Olivia's body and showing her husband how to discover what kinds of touch turned her on, she sat up from the massage table with huge tears in her eyes. Her husband stood there lovingly with his hand on her back.

I could feel the confidence flooding into him.

"I've waited twenty years to be touched like that." She patted her eyes with the tissue I handed her. "Maybe I've waited my whole life to be touched like that!" She sobbed tears of joy.

Her husband held her with deep presence and love. "You just saved our marriage!" she exclaimed.

We helped her down from the table the moment her wobbly legs felt like they could stand again. "I've never experienced anything like that. I was so present and in my body!" Olivia was in awe after her body-mapping session.

I was once again in awe myself. The rewards of this experience are always powerful.

While I don't believe I can save anyone or their relationships—it's the willingness to learn and do the work that is their saving grace, not me—I do believe in the power of loving presence and loving, attuned touch to connect people and make them feel seen and cherished. I do believe the conscious practice of these skills can transform people and their relationships. Hands-on practice will give you the skills and experience needed for increased pleasure and satisfaction.

Olivia had just had the experience of her husband being there for her with deep presence, learning how to be more skillful in his touch and how to play her body the way it liked to be played best. In some ways, that was a small miracle, and this practice can "save" relationships.

Combining Body Mapping and the A/B Game

Now that you've learned the A/B game and body mapping, it's time to combine them for an advanced experience that gives you more specific embodied information.

You'll need all the same tools as mentioned earlier in this chapter, but a longer amount of time to work within. When I'm working with a couple in my practice, we spend a whole day mapping both partners. Each person receives a three-hour combined mapping session with a lunch break in between. It's an amazing way to spend a day. If you're working solo, you will want to set aside at least three hours to go through your entire body, head to toe, with this deeper-level exploration. Couples should set aside six hours with a lunchtime break to complete their sessions.

Begin by choosing the order in which you would like to explore the Erotic Blueprints. For example, you may want to begin with your Primary

Blueprint, or with information you discovered during an earlier A/B game or body-mapping session. You may also be curious about specific parts of your body. For example, you might try doing a deeper session mapping your genitals with all the different Blueprint Touches.

The premise is the same. You will rate sensations on a scale of 1 to 5 and then use the A/B game to go deeper.

Here are some ways to explore if you're doing this on your own.

Begin by using an Energetic touch stroke with light fingertips up your inner thigh; as you touch, practice meeting sensation with awareness and breath. After thirty seconds or so of touch, ask yourself how pleasurable this is on a scale of 1 to 5. Rate the sensation.

Choose who will give and receive first. Then play with the following elements:

» Speed: Go faster or slower
» Location: Make the stroke longer or shorter
» Depth: Give more or less pressure
» Sensation: Add an additional stimulus

As you incorporate each of these elements, ask yourself if this increases or decreases pleasure. Ultimately, this is a different way of saying A or B— you're looking more for what increases or decreases pleasure.

Here's an example of how to do this with a partner.

Imagine you are the giver in this scenario. Massage your partner with warm oil, starting from their foot and moving up to their hip with medium pressure and contoured touch. Ask them, "On a scale of one to five, how pleasurable is this?" You can then change the speed, depth of pressure, or location (with longer or shorter strokes) of the touch, or add another sensation to what you just tried. Note their response.

Keep exploring in the same area with variations to see what turns them on most. When you are changing the sensation, guide your partner verbally by stating what you're modifying; for example, "Here is faster" or "Here is slower."

Ask your partner which touch they prefer, and repeat the touch if they have a hard time deciding. Of course, they're allowed to like them both equally!

At the end of the session, express your gratitude to each other and talk about what worked. If you are solo, this is a great time to write what you learned about yourself in a journal.

Troubleshooting When Things Go South (and Not in a Good Way)

Sometimes, an A/B game or body-mapping session doesn't go as planned. Perhaps your partner got angry partway through and stopped the exercise. Or maybe they felt nothing, or didn't experience much pleasure. Perhaps you got impatient and wanted to end the exercise before it even started. Or maybe one of the touch sensations triggered an unsettling emotional response in you. Maybe one of you had a rough day—or was tired, or had gas, or had a bad day at work, or felt overwhelmed with stress. Maybe something had shifted in your body. Maybe your fingernails were scratchy but your partner wasn't speaking up. The list goes on and on . . .

Research indicates that people with higher levels of the stress hormone cortisol tend to experience lower levels of sexual desire, sexual activity, sexual satisfaction, and sexual pleasure. This increase in cortisol can occur due to accumulated daily stress or stressful life events. Over time, this has been shown to negatively impact relationships.

So many factors can change our receptivity to pleasure, so it's important not to think you have it all figured out or know everything now.

My response to any of these scenarios is: Don't. Give. Up. If you're committed to your Blueprint journey, you should be able to find a way to work through—and recover from—any disappointment or discomfort. Here are some ways to do so.

TRY THINGS MORE THAN ONCE. Play with these exercises at least three times before you give it the thumbs-up or thumbs-down. Many factors can affect how you experience any type of touch. For example, where are you on your hormonal cycle, or how was your blood sugar the day you did the practice? Did you and your partner have a disagreement beforehand? Or did you simply not give yourself enough time?

DON'T TAKE ANYTHING PERSONALLY. Part of learning is getting feedback. If you get defensive and take your partner's feedback critically, you've lost the game. Can you let go of your ego and look at your expansion into pleasure as a practice or a hobby, instead of a competition? You aren't playing the game to get it right or to "win." You're playing the game to have fun, discover more pleasure, and find juicy fulfillment.

If you're the one giving the feedback, stay positive and don't criticize your partner. You are learning together.

IGNORE YOUR INNER CRITIC. Quiet the voices in your head that whisper you aren't doing it right, or that you are not good enough because you have to do this on your own. If it helps, choose a positive phrase to repeat as you're doing the exercises. Something like "I am love" or "I am pleasured."

Don't fret if you try some of what you learned and take it into your sexual play (I hope you do!), but find that the techniques are not quite as pleasurable this time. You can't expect everything to be pleasurable every time. And mastery of anything takes practice, so don't pressure yourself or your partner to have it perfect right away.

CONNECT WITH EXPERTS AND FIND A WELCOMING COMMUNITY. Having a community of sex-positive and informed supporters can help you stay on track and break through the blocks of societal programming. Seeing other people working through the same challenges helps end the isolation that can keep you stuck. Suddenly you'll see that you are not alone or unique in your challenges, and this can be profoundly healing. It can also give you a sense of freedom as you collectively strive to discover the truth about sex and who you are in relationship to that truth.

See the resources section (page 287) for information on how to connect with communities and experts who can help you on your journey of sexual self-discovery. Play nice, please!

Keep these factors in mind, but whatever you do, don't blame an unsuccessful body-mapping session on your perceived sexual incompatibly. It's time to put that to bed, because in the next chapter, I'm going to tell you exactly how Erotic Blueprint Types play together.

CHAPTER THIRTEEN

how blueprints play together

The TV show host leaned in as if she was asking me to tell her a secret. "What do we do when we have different Erotic Blueprints and want different things when it comes to our sex lives?" It's a frequent question, and I rarely escape an interview without it being asked. In fact, I've heard this question so often over the years that at this point, I have a succinct answer ready to go: Be willing to learn how to feed and speak each other's Blueprints.

But since this is a book, not TV, I'm going to spend some time going into detail about how each Blueprint pairing likes to play together.

The first thing to understand when it comes to pairing different Blueprint Types is that each pair has both merits and drawbacks. If you and your partner are willing to learn each other's Erotic Blueprints, a lot of expansion can happen for everyone!

I'll say it again: Even if it seems like you are mismatched, you aren't doomed—you just need to be patient and open to learning. And you may even find that your opposing desires can actually work to both of your benefit—you just need to learn how.

Pleasure First: Opposites Integrate

Lay down flat on your back with your knees in the air.

Place one hand on your heart and the other on your genitals. You can think of the hand on your heart as connecting with the Energetic Blueprint and the hand on your genitals as connecting with the Sexual Blueprint.

First, feel the hand on your heart and feel into the Energetic Blueprint. Allow yourself to feel it fully. Notice images, thoughts, body sensations, and emotions that arise.

Now put your awareness on the hand on your genitals, and feel into the Sexual Blueprint. Allow the thoughts, images, body sensation, and emotions to arise and notice them as they do.

Once again put your awareness on the hand at your heart. Lean into the images, thoughts, body sensations, and emotions that arise as you feel into the Energetic Blueprint. You can begin to make small circles with your hand, adding stimulation.

Again put your awareness on the hand at your genitals and feel into the Sexual Blueprint. Add any stimulation that feels good here. Intensify the images, emotions, thoughts, and body sensations.

Repeat one more time with each hand.

Now feel both the heart (Energetic) and the genitals (Sexual) at the same time. Take a deep breath, feeling them both at the same time. As you exhale and feel them simultaneously, notice what happens.

Continue this practice until the two have become one or everything just becomes blank and there are no more images, thoughts, body sensations, or emotions. There is usually a great pleasure when they come into union with each other.

Embody It: Finding Your Erotic Bridges

Create an uninterrupted space and time to sit with your partner. You will need a journal to write responses in.

If you do not have a lover, I highly recommend doing this exercise for yourself anyway so you'll know the depth of what you would like to explore with any future partners.

Close your eyes and hold hands. Breathe together.

Open your eyes and connect for a moment, putting your attention on each other. Hold the idea that anything is possible while you gaze directly into your lover's left eye. Soften your gaze.

Take five minutes here (which will feel like an eternity to some of you) to hold unconditional love for each other. Remind yourself that there is nothing to be fixed, nothing they need to be or do for you to love them.

Keep breathing, and feel the love and connection you have for each other.

Then begin this dyad. We did this exercise earlier in the book with different prompts. Remember that in a dyad you and your partner give the same prompt back and forth until you complete the exercise.

Your prompt for this dyad is: Tell me something you think would feed both of us sexually.

After you or your partner responds to the prompt, the other can give one of four responses:

» Thank you.
» Say it again.
» Clarify that.
» Summarize that.

Take a moment to write down each answer that is stated. Whoever gives the prompt should be the writer. (Or you can use a voice recorder instead.)

After twenty minutes of this dyad, you should have a pretty good list of ideas.

Make a copy of the list so you each have one. Sitting separately and apart from each other, circle all the activities that you are interested in exploring on your copy of the list, and cross out any activities that you aren't interested in. Now, look at the ones you circled, and put a check mark next to those you're willing to explore and an exclamation point next to the ones you definitely want to explore.

Then come together and compare your lists.

Anything that you both "want to" or are "willing to" explore can go on your exploration list.

Now it's time to prioritize your to-do list.

Make a plan together to start to implement those ideas. Perhaps designate a set time each week to explore something on your list. Anything you both responded to with an exclamation point should be first on your to-do list, since those are what I would call "easy wins."

Willingness Is a Must

I say this again and again, but what holds most people back from attaining the sexual life they desire is a resistance to personal growth and an unwillingness to learn new skills. We often hold on to limiting belief systems that we have acquired throughout our lives.

Being resistant makes it very difficult for anyone to help you. If you're unwilling to learn the skills to please your partner, you're at a dead end. This behavior is the number one reason relationships stay stuck. If you don't believe that anything will work for you, this belief will eventually become a self-fulfilling prophecy.

Are you trying to avoid something deeper that's going on? Are you running away from pain? Are there buried resentments you don't wish to confront or believe your partner is unwilling to address? Does intimacy of this kind terrify you?

These can be difficult questions to ask yourself and your partner, but they can also be incredibly rewarding to explore.

It can be challenging to work through this on your own, but a great sexuality or Erotic Blueprint coach, therapist, or sex-positive couples counselor can help you if you feel stuck.

When we work through the resistance, we begin to bridge the gaps between our erotic desires, which gets us closer to building lasting relationships. Finding your Erotic Bridges is a golden ticket to an unending world of discovery and possibility in your erotic life.

How Erotic Blueprints Play Together and Stay Together

Curiosity breeds intimacy, and the more we understand our lover(s), the more we are able to understand ourselves and our needs within that relationship.

Once you know your Erotic Blueprint Types, you can learn how your pairing best plays together so that you can flourish on a foundation of love and prioritize pleasure in your relationship.

ENERGETIC WITH ENERGETIC

Two Energetics together can truly have out-of-this-world and out-of-this-body sex! They can deeply feel each other. They go infinitely slow together. Their orgasms can be mutual Energetic dances in cosmic realms.

On the flip side, feeling everything can lead to a lack of physical sexual connection. If there is any dissociation, the Energetics may check out during sex or have difficulty connecting in the physical world. Not connecting in the physical isn't a bad thing, unless one of the Energetics has a strong secondary in another Blueprint that needs attention, or there is more desire from one partner to have a more Sexual relationship.

One of my lovers and I dance in this dynamic. He is a gay man (I know, it's confusing—it was for us, too—and yes, he still identifies as a gay, and yes, we are erotic together). My first big Tantric awakenings happened in his arms. And in twenty years together, we haven't had physical intercourse.

We have also had a lot of confusion and a lot of pain as we tried to navigate understanding our connection. For many years, we struggled because my Sexual aspect couldn't believe that he loved me if we weren't having intercourse.

It took us a good seventeen years to come to the realization and acceptance that the Energetic Blueprint was the foundation of our relationship. We eventually found an authentic pathway to express our boundless hearts. Things between us are highly erotic energetically; we just didn't meet in the Sexual Blueprint.

Just being in proximity to each other, we start to vibrate on a frequency unlike anything I have ever had with any other Blueprint combination.

Wow, can we travel!

So if you're dancing in this dynamic, it may be time to accept that your connection is more energetic and spiritual, and not meant to be sexual in this lifetime. Get clear on what you need, and if you do need a more physical sexual life, you'll want to see where you can bridge more or have a conversation about getting your physical needs met by opening your relationship to other lovers. You may find ways that are not Sexual Blueprint to feel more connected in the physical world, spending time practicing Tantra together, for example, or going to a sound bath together.

ENERGETIC WITH SENSUAL

Energetics and Sensuals play very well together in that they both appreciate safety and having a beautiful environment they play in. They can go slow together, they can delight in each other, and both enjoy deliciously slow, light touches, kisses, and lovemaking.

On the Shadow side, these two may find themselves in an endless battle around physical space. The Energetic wants space, and the Sensual lights up when space collapses—physical closeness is their turn-on. When this dynamic isn't understood, it often results in a runner/chaser dynamic. The Sensual is usually chasing the Energetic, while the Energetic isn't turned on and may even become distressed when there isn't enough space for them to feel.

Ian loves to collapse the space between us. Dancing with our bodies entwined, massage, cuddling close, lying on top of me, these are just some of his favorite ways to feel connected. If we're having a moment of disagreement, he wants to come closer, and I want space.

Often this would get so intense for me that I would physically run out of the space we were in before I exploded emotionally and said things I didn't want to say. If he kept pursuing me, I would say, "I'm done!" (with an energy of "I'm leaving you!"). It was an ugly run-and-chase dynamic rooted in both of our Erotic Blueprints.

Bringing awareness to the dynamic was the first step toward finding a solution. It was also important for me to better recognize when I needed to ask Ian for space and reassure him that I wasn't leaving and would be available to cuddle after I had had space and time to calm down. That worked like a charm.

If you find yourself in an Energetic/Sensual dynamic, gaining some clarity on both of your relationships with physical space is a useful step. Getting the space you need may be an aspect of your relationship that requires careful negotiation.

ENERGETIC WITH SEXUAL

This pairing has a lot to teach each other. They are in many ways polar opposites, but that's one of the beauties of this relationship.

The Energetic slows down the Sexual and teaches them how to be present in the moment. An Energetic can introduce a Sexual to the spiritual side of sex, broadening their experience to include things they didn't imagine were possible or were even a part of intimacy to begin with.

The Sexual can ground the Energetic into the wondrous pleasures of physical sex and the body.

But sometimes the challenges this pairing faces can feel truly insurmountable.

The Sexual can have a very hard time understanding how anyone can feel pleasure if they aren't having their body or genitals touched. They can get very impatient and angry, especially when they're having to slow down and learn the skills needed to please their Energetic lover.

The Energetic can get very judgmental of the Sexual and lose compassion for their partner. Oftentimes the Energetic feels their Sexual partner doesn't honor their personal boundaries, body, and sensitivities. The Energetic may have continually overridden their needs to please the Sexual and then begun to blame their Sexual partner for the tension or resentment they feel.

For this pairing to work, it's important for both partners to be patient and to take the time to learn skills that truly please each other, without the resentment that sometimes comes with having to learn something new. Seek to understand each other. The Energetic needs to understand their Sexual partner's point of view, and how their deep need to have sex is equally as important as our basic need for love, food, air, or water. The Sexual needs to understand the traumas and negative experiences that created the high sensitivity that Energetics experience and that often results in their intense need for slowness and space. These are keys for deeper connection and positive expansion in a loving relationship.

Liam and Charlotte were caught deep in the Shadows of their respective Blueprints. Liam wanted sex all the time. Charlotte wanted different sex than the sex they were having. Liam loved Charlotte's body and wanted to touch her and have sex with her every day. If he didn't ejaculate and have intercourse, his tension would build until it became so strong, he felt it was Charlotte's "duty" to take care of him. He couldn't understand why she had to be in a certain "space" to have sex.

Charlotte, on the other hand, was tired of being "mauled" all the time. She wanted foreplay and lots of time to warm up to intercourse, but she felt he didn't really care about her or how she felt, that he just wanted to "put it in" and then "pump until he was satisfied" with no regard for her pleasure. Her body was screaming no, and yet she would lie there and allow the pattern to continue. She felt like an object, there to serve his needs. She didn't want to face his disappointment if she said no. She didn't want to feel his increasing tension if she didn't have sex with him.

Luckily, Liam was very willing to learn new skills. He actually wanted to please his wife; he had just been so caught up in relieving his tension that he wasn't aware of the harm being created between them. With awareness of his own body and then of his wife's, he could see what was really going on. They weren't having the sex he wanted, either.

Charlotte learned how to speak up, gain agency, and ask him to slow down and give her space when she needed it. She was highly orgasmic; she just needed the breathing room to feel all the pleasure coursing through her body. Eventually, she learned the joy of her body and her pleasure through Liam's hands, mouth, and genitals.

If you are in this dynamic, not to worry. If you're both willing to learn and to have compassion (and to stop trying to fix each other), there's no limit to the pleasure you can find together. Expanding your Blueprint will be a huge help—I'll cover that more in chapter sixteen.

ENERGETIC WITH KINKY

Energetics and Kinkys can play very well together, especially if the Kinky is very psychological and enjoys activities such as role-playing. The two can find many realms to explore, including Dom/sub space, power games, and expanded states of awareness. There can be endless fun, dimensions, and realms to play in.

However, if the Energetic is caught in the Shadow of judgment and feeling superior to other Blueprints, they will deeply judge and misunderstand the Kinky. The Kinky will often go into a shame spiral as a result, and will begin to hide who they are as an erotic being. This can create a lot of disconnection between them.

Also, if the Kinky loves impact play and some of the edgier sensation-based spaces, this can intimidate the Energetic, who may be reluctant to play there—especially if they tend to fall more on the lighter, more spiritual side of their Blueprint.

My clients Christy and Nathan struggled with this particular dynamic. Nathan liked to play within kink, but Christy felt turned off by the edgier things he wanted to explore. They needed some bridges between their Blueprints. In working with me, they found that teasing and edging Christy energetically until she couldn't stand it anymore pleased both of them. She would beg for Nathan to ground her with some physical touch. He loved playing with this energy, and she loved how it lit him up! They had found a bridge between their Kinky and Energetic turn-ons, and it was so hot.

If you are in this dynamic, working through places of shame for the Kinky or judgment from the Energetic is the first area to start. Creating healthy boundaries and having careful negotiations will help you both discover which realms are available for you to explore together.

ENERGETIC WITH SHAPESHIFTER

This pairing is wonderful because both Blueprints can dance together as Energetics.

What is unique here is that the Shapeshifter can take the Energetic to many different realms within the Energetic. It's quite magical to see this happen. The best way I can describe it is that the Shapeshifter will move through all the Blueprints, but do so energetically. The Energetic brings out this Superpower in the Shapeshifter.

But the Shapeshifter needs to be very aware of getting their more physical needs met. This is a risk for the Shapeshifter with any Blueprint they are paired with. Are they Shapeshifting to meet the needs of their lover but, in turn, not getting their own needs met?

The Energetic may become easily overwhelmed by the Shapeshifter and can move into short-circuiting or dissociating. This can be very challenging for the Shapeshifter, who wants to keep playing but feels their lover is no longer present with them.

James, Theo, and Harper—a poly triad—had a pretty good sex life when they came to work with me. James, an Energetic, was navigating two very vibrant Shapeshifters and had begun to feel overwhelmed by all the energy and the length of their play sessions as a triad. It seemed that Theo and Harper could go for hours and hours, but there would come a time when James would just "poop out." At that point he would also "pop out" of his body. Theo would feel abandoned because it was like James wasn't there with them anymore. Harper would start to chase the waning turn-on, making it worse for everyone.

The simple solution was to give James breaks in their play sessions and to help him assimilate all the erotic energy. In these moments, Theo and Harper could play together, and James could breathe. When one of them played alone with James, it was important to ground him at times so that he could drop back into his body. James eventually learned how to increase his capacity to play with his two Shapeshifter lovers. And because his lovers knew how to ground him and give him rest, he could fly way out in the cosmos and be in his body at the same time.

If you are in a Shapeshifter/Energetic relationship, sit down together and talk about what will help the Energetic assimilate all the energy and sensation from the Shapeshifter so they don't get overwhelmed. You may want to revisit the section of the book where I talk about assimilation tools (see pages 107–108). And Energetics, look at ways you can increase your capacity for physical pleasure so that you feel less overwhelmed during sex. Before you know it, you'll be going on marathons with your Shapeshifter lover(s)!

SENSUAL WITH SENSUAL

Two Sensuals together are like a soup of deliciousness with flavors that delight the tongue. They are a snugglefest, bodies entwined in sensuous dance. When two Sensuals are together, they create the sexiest boudoir ever imagined. Sensuals can fall into each other's bodies and find a never-ending playground of delights.

However, when caught in the Shadow together, two Sensuals can become a hypervigilant nightmare. Nothing is ever right. Nothing can ever be right. There's never enough time for lovemaking or deliciousness. There's so much stress and tension in life, and it gets in the way of the "mood," if the mood ever arises to begin with. Sensuals do not know how to relax enough to reach the amazing wonders of themselves, and they miss each other and the unending pleasure possibilities.

Mia and Sophia were so very alike (their names even rhymed!). Both were very sophisticated and successful. But as full-time entrepreneurs in a shared design business, they found themselves sorely lacking in sensual connection. They were both creatives but spent all their time creating wondrous spaces for others, not with or for each other.

Mia had a very hard time transitioning from work to being present with Sophia each day. Since they owned a business together, it was easy to fall back into work discussions at home when they were supposed to be sharing a romantic time. They both expected the mood to arise naturally. When it didn't, they blamed each other, which created even more stress. They were in a self-defeating loop.

We created easy toggles that allowed them to let go of work at the end of the day and maintain boundaries around their work schedule; for example, they would take turns setting up a hot herbal bath for each other. They both needed transitions into the sensuous realm, and they needed to stop expecting it to just arise naturally. This was a big first step for the couple toward creating a relaxed, timeless space of their own, where they could be fully present with each other's bodies.

For you and your Sensual lover, it's time to make space for yourselves. What can you do in your environment to make your lovemaking space more inviting? What transitions do you need to let go of the world and just be in your body? Start making time with your like-minded partner. Encourage each other to create boundaries between your erotic lives and everything else. Additionally, take time together to create a sumptuous space for sensuality.

SENSUAL WITH SEXUAL

The good news is that both the Sensual and the Sexual love bodies—being in their bodies, playing with bodies, touching bodies. Making love to bodies is especially enjoyable together. This pair can get lost in lovemaking together, and that's a wonderful thing.

The challenge here is that the Sensual loves long, slow buildups that do not necessarily have any clear goal or direction. The Sexual, on the other hand, loves the certainty that genital stimulation, intercourse, and orgasm are going to happen. This can feel like pressure to the Sensual, sending them into their heads and simply turning them off.

The Sexual may also miss the artistry of the experience, focusing too much on the end goal and not enough on foreplay, sensation play, or creating a beautiful environment for their lover. The Sexual, in their desire to relieve their own tension through sex, can miss that the Sensual needs to relieve tension too before they can relax into great sex.

Harper and Lucas were really struggling when they came for their immersion. Harper could not understand why it was so hard for Lucas to just have sex. Lucas complained that all Harper cared about was getting to the orgasm and didn't know how to pleasure him at all.

We spent our first day together focusing on Lucas. Harper learned to slow down and to create safety and a beautiful space. She learned to listen and be in the present experience of feeling sensation. On the second day, it was Harper's turn, and we learned just how much of a sexual appetite she had. It was hard for her to receive touch and sensuality; it felt very intimate and vulnerable. The day was fulfilling, and a stretch emotionally.

By day three, they were already finding bridges, like slow dancing naked, skin to skin. A week later, they were having fulfilling and frequent sex, and it was better than it had ever been. All it took was some learning and opening themselves to some new approaches, which they were both willing to do.

If you are in a Sensual/Sexual match, it's important to realize that you both love playing in the body. For the Sexual, it's time to slow down, listen, and attune to your Sensual lover. Learn new skills that involve pleasuring the whole body, not just the primary erogenous zones.

For the Sensual, realize that your Sexual lover *loves* sex, and that they most likely want to have sex with you anytime. Ask your Sexual lover for touch that isn't about getting to the end goal, but just about enjoyment of each other. And use your toggles and transitions to help you get into a sexual space if you want to have your fire burning for them before they even initiate sex.

SENSUAL WITH KINKY

These two are all about sensation, sensation, sensation when they play together. The Sensual/Kinky world is filled with experiential delights. This pairing has a huge variety of ways to play together, especially if the Kinky is more sensation-oriented.

The Kinky can help the Sensual get out of their head by providing a more intense sensation-based experience. The meeting place for these two lies in creativity, full-body play together, and, of course, sensation!

The Kinky can test the capacity of the Sensual, if the Kinky is into a lot of impact and/or more intense sensation play. This may lead the Sensual to shut down, which in turn can send the Kinky into a shame spiral about their desires. If both partners prefer to be on the receiving end of sensation rather than giving it, difficulties can arise. If the Sensual is unwilling to learn what turns on the Kinky in their realm, it can create shame and distance, and provoke the Kinky to hide their desires.

Rich and Kelly were in a new relationship.

Only a month in, and Kelly was shocked to discover that Rich was Kinky. She wasn't at all familiar with kink and even had many false assumptions about people who were Kinky. When the couple turned their focus to Kelly's Sensual Blueprint, the sex was great. She felt seen for the first time in a relationship, and the sex was so slow and sensuous.

But Rich was feeling left out. He loved pleasing her, but he knew that given more time, things wouldn't last if he didn't reveal his desires.

At the six-month mark, Kelly reached out for help.

She was willing to learn about kink, but had no idea where to begin. She was intimidated by Rich's desires and enjoyed the receiving role most, so giving to him felt forced. Luckily, through time and lots of classes and resources, she was able to gain more confidence and skill at pleasing Rich. They also realized together that creating a great sex life is an ongoing process. I'm pleased to say that they are still happy students six years later and are committed to a lifetime of learning.

If you're in a Kinky/Sensual pairing, you may find yourself relying a lot on the sensuous nature of your relationship, but it may be time to learn more about what is possible, especially when it comes to the desires and delights of the Kinky's realm.

Take a course together, hire a kink expert to show you the ropes (pun intended), and make a commitment to sexual mastery for as long as you are in the relationship.

SENSUAL WITH SHAPESHIFTER

What is so wonderful here is that the Shapeshifter and the Sensual, like the Shapeshifter and the Kinky, can dance deliciously in the realms of everything sensation-based. There can be a lot of variety in their erotic expression, and they can utilize a lot of erotic creativity together.

But as I've mentioned, a Shapeshifter's kryptonite is that they shift to please their partner and eventually find themselves starving. Sensuals can find themselves easily overwhelmed by the Shapeshifter's agility, and will feel the stress of performance anxiety in the face of the Shapeshifter's need for variety and more, more, more. This can leave the Shapeshifter in the Shadow; once again feeling like they are too much, they shrink their erotic intelligence to fit a more bite-size mold.

Donald and Barb were completing their forty-fourth year together. Their goal was to make it to their fiftieth wedding anniversary with a passionate sex life. In recent years, they had found themselves drifting apart in the bedroom. Barb complained that their sex life was getting stale and lacking in variety. Donald found himself wanting more cuddling and less sexual intercourse. The issues Barb and Donald outlined are only to be expected after forty-four years together, and I was proud of them for their desire to keep their sexual relationship alive.

They were still mad about each other—they just needed a little boost.

Donald had moved into more of a Resting Sensual Blueprint as he was getting older, and his testosterone levels were lower than in previous years. He was grateful for this, as he felt he could relax more into sex than ever before. But his go-to had become cuddling and kissing and maybe going down on Barb when he had more energy.

Barb, a true Shapeshifter, was still going strong, with a vivacious libido and lovely appetite for creative sexual play. She was having her own sexual renaissance and claimed she felt more confident than she ever had when she was younger.

Donald received some hormonal support that boosted his testosterone. With revived energy, he and Barb were ready to go on a new sexual adventure together. They were retired, so they had plenty of time to devote to their adventures. I suggested they start going on retreats to explore a different Blueprint each month.

Together they went on to explore Tantra, which Donald discovered he had a knack for, and Bondassage, a hybrid of massage and kink. They began to learn more advanced sex skills, such as G-spot and prostate massage. And they were thrilled to find out that after forty-four years, they had so much more to discover about each other. Their relationship blossomed, and they found that there is no end to what they can explore, as long as they both stay willing.

If you are in a Sensual/Shapeshifter pairing, it's time to spice things up by finding a variety of ways you can play together. Make sure you don't get trapped in the comfort zones of the Sensual, and that you bring in more variety and adventure for the Shapeshifter.

SEXUAL WITH SEXUAL

Well, here's a hot pair! Can't keep their hands off each other. You might find them fucking at any time, day or night!

Two Sexuals together *love* to have lots of sex, in lots of positions, with lots of getting right to the main event! Skip the meal—let's just have dessert!

The challenge with two Sexuals together is that like a blazing fire, they can burn out quickly. The spark is there, then suddenly, out it goes. They can also have a very hard time when life changes or health changes arise, because they don't know any other way to connect.

Oftentimes when we describe a couple as having great sexual chemistry, it's two Sexuals together. But sexual chemistry doesn't equal a great relationship, and I see a lot of people who stay in relationships that aren't good for them, or even downright toxic, because of their sexual chemistry.

Adrianna knew her "boyfriend" Steve wasn't good for her at all. He was like a drug, and that drug had really bad side effects in her life.

Steve was verbally abusive, and he had cheated on Adrianna more than once. Yet when he would call her drunk late at night, her whole body would light up with arousal. Adrianna began to work with her therapist to unravel why it was so hard for her to stop the unhealthy cycle of enabling him to mistreat her. She did the hard work of starting to say no and to make healthier choices for herself. And with awareness of the other Blueprints, she could see that dating another Sexual wasn't the best choice for her, at least not until she had healed and learned to put her physical and mental health first.

Eventually, she found a lover who was a Primary Sexual but unlike Steve, still treated her with love and respect. He was also willing to tap into other Blueprints, which would allow their relationship to adapt as life brought changes or the "chemistry" wore off, giving them longevity.

What helps this pairing keep passion alive? A first step is recognizing the potential for the relationship to become toxic and identifying destructive behaviors. Healing the Shadow sides that may involve unhealthy behaviors leaves room for deepening growth. Eventually, you may need to expand into other Blueprint pleasures. High libido can shift throughout life. That initial passion can fade, so having other Blueprints to feed your eroticism is key. Be prepared to expand your erotic intelligence and incorporate variety into your sexual play.

SEXUAL WITH KINKY

When these two are on together, they are on!

The Sexual/Kinky pairing can be unique and very surprising. Together they can play in all the naughty realms, and the Kinky inspires the Sexual to get much more creative.

The challenge with this pairing is that the Kinky needs a lot more variety than the Sexual does. The Sexual can feel annoyed by the complexity of kinky play, and the Kinky can feel bored and rushed as a result. If the Sexual is unable or unwilling to meet the desires of the Kinky, the Kinky may feel shame, as well as a sense of defeat at the thought that their needs will never be met.

It was the biggest eye roll I'd ever seen from a Sexual. I had simply suggested that Harold slow down when tying up his lover Sam. The ties were Sam's request. "It takes so loooooong," Harold moaned. "I'm fumbling with ropes instead of fucking. And it's boring. I can't keep my erection at all."

"Who said you had to keep an erection? And who are the ropes for?" I asked, challenging him a bit. I understood his pain, but this was the Sexual Shadow showing up, an unwillingness to meet the wants and needs of his partner. Unfortunately, Harold remained resistant and unwilling to meet Sam's needs, and unwilling to try or to learn anything new. The sex dwindled to nothing, and the relationship ended.

Playing in this pairing, as with all these pairings, just takes a willingness to learn what turns each other on and to find the bridges between you and your partner. Don't be like Harold.

The Sexual needs to be open to—and patient with—the desires of the Kinky. The Kinky can come to understand that sometimes getting right to it or handing over the reins to the Sexual can be the hottest part of the power play!

SEXUAL WITH SHAPESHIFTER

As with other Shapeshifter pairings, the ability to play in the same Blueprint makes this bedroom dynamic wonderful.

In the Shadow dance of these two, the Sexual can get super rigid and find the needs of the Shapeshifter either boring or too much to deal with.

The Sexual digs their heels in and gets turned off by taking so much time to play the way the Shapeshifter desires. As usual, the Shapeshifter may find themself shapeshifting to please their Sexual partner and then starving and building resentment in return.

This pair has the biggest Sexual appetite of all the pairings, especially if one of them happens to also be a Sexual Shapeshifter. If they both love to go for hours and hours, multiple times a day, they may find themselves not getting anything done!

Keith, a bisexual Shapeshifter in his forties, loved dating couples.

One couple he enjoyed playing with was especially Sexual, and he really enjoyed himself when he was with them. After a while, however, the sex started to feel the same each time he played with them. No appetizer, a little bit of dinner, right to dessert, then good night and to sleep.

As he began to learn about the Erotic Blueprints, Keith came to understand why the sex felt boring to him: He was a Shapeshifter, and he needed a lot more variety than what was being offered. He shared with the couple that he would love to do some more creative play. He got out the massage table and invited them to tie him to it, then massage him and use sensation toys. They could also play with each other while they played with him.

It worked!

Keith was elated that by realizing he was a Primary Shapeshifter, he came to understand a lot about himself and felt empowered to ask for the time, variety, and creativity he so longed for.

Be like Keith and his lovers! If you are a Shapeshifter paired with a Sexual, it's time to tell them you want more variety, more play, more, more, more. As your partner learns, be compassionate and patient with them. Realize that all this desire for more may be overwhelming, frustrating, or boring to them.

And Sexuals, it's okay to ask for your needs to be met, too. At a bare minimum, your Shapeshifter should feed you with a quickie now and then.

KINKY WITH KINKY

Yummy, taboo for two!

One Kinky alone is an endless world of exploration; two adds the potential for boundless creativity.

The challenge with the Kinky/Kinky dynamic lies in who is turned on by what. Do you have two Kinky people who both want to be submissive? Do you have two Kinky people who both want to play the puppy trainer, not the puppy?

Katy and Fae both tested high for the Kinky Blueprint. The issue was not that they didn't want to learn together or that they came from different worlds. It was that they both wanted the same thing. Fae wanted to be in the submissive role, to be a service submissive. Katy, too, wanted to be the receiver and the submissive. This left no one to play the Dominant role.

When they came to this realization, they understood why things between them had fallen flat. They were both waiting for the other to take the reins and initiate a scene. They were very new to kink and young to their own sexuality, so they hadn't explored themselves much, but as they came to know each other and what they were turned on by, it became clear that there was a challenge.

Lucky for them, they had a foundation of love to grow on. We discovered that they were both willing to take turns being the giver/receiver or Dominant/submissive. They were both willing to learn and to expand their turn-ons so they could play together. Both still find the most turn-on when they get to be the one in submission, but now they have a lot more versatility.

If you are paired Kinky/Kinky and want to play in different roles, this may be no issue for you, especially if you are open and willing to learn how to meet your lover's desires. If, however, you and your partner are like Fae and Katy, you may want to expand and discuss how you both can switch it up a bit.

KINKY WITH SHAPESHIFTER

Whoever is paired with a Shapeshifter is likely to find their needs met.

In general, Shapeshifter and Kinky pairs play well together because they both thrive in creative erotic environments. Most Shapeshifters will not shame a Kinky person or find their desires intimidating because they also have taboo desires and understand on some level what their Kinky partner is feeling. And when it comes to sex, this pair likes marathon sessions.

The Kinky, like the other Blueprints, may feel that the Shapeshifter is too much. There may be an apparent mismatch in other Blueprints with the Shapeshifter, for example, if the Shapeshifter has a lot of Energetic Shadow. They may pass judgment on their Kinky partner, or find them completely overwhelming; there may be distance inside this relationship.

Lailah and Jordan felt like they were running a sexual marathon each time they had sex. Jordan loved the Kinky scenes that Lailah would create; they were so creative and thoughtful. Lailah would surprise Jordan by having the bedroom set up as a Kinky playroom, and they would do elaborate scenes with role-play, costumes and all.

Jordan, however, was getting tired, while Lailah felt she wasn't getting enough sex. They had a huge aha moment when they realized that Jordan was Kinky and Lailah was a Shapeshifter. Instantly, Jordan went to work creating extravagant experiences for Lailah that included all the Blueprints, while Lailah began to indulge in the art of satiation, a practice for feeling satisfied and being able to sit with your desire for more and more and more.

Their love deepened as each could see just how much the other cared for and wanted to please them.

If you are in a Kinky/Shapeshifter pairing, it can be fun to set up different kinds of scenes for each other. These could be Kinky role-play sessions or extravagant scenes where the Shapeshifter gets to play in all the flavors.

SHAPESHIFTER WITH SHAPESHIFTER

Whoa! I'm in awe of this pairing. They have infinite ways to enjoy every single Blueprint.

Creativity is through the roof, through the cosmos, through the body, through it all! They want to pleasure each other and be pleasured for hours on end. They can. They do.

The biggest challenge with this dynamic is that if they both shapeshift all over the place, they may never be on the same page on the same night. One wants to play Kinky, but the other is all Energetic. One wants Sexual, but the other is Sensual. Each night becomes about bridging gaps, which may lead to lots of frustration instead of sexy time.

Bo and Mic loved sex, loved to play, loved to pleasure and be pleasured. Both wanted more, because neither of them felt satisfied. One issue was that their skills didn't match their desires. They wanted to play with kink, they wanted to do Tantra, they wanted all the things, but they didn't know how to do them effectively, safely, or with any level of mastery. That was an easy shift—all they had to do was learn.

At a deeper level, however, it wasn't just about learning: Bo and Mic were shapeshifting to different places without consciously knowing it had happened. When Bo was Sexual, Mic would get very Energetic and run away, wanting space. When Mic went Sexual, Bo would go Sensual and want to cuddle instead. Their wires kept getting crossed.

We solved this by scheduling three-hour chunks for them to play with full-on Shapeshifter experiences. There was no rush; they could get fed in every Blueprint, and no one would starve! And most important, neither had to chase the pleasure they craved.

If you're in a Shapeshifter/Shapeshifter pairing, don't leave any Blueprint out when it comes to your erotic time together. Learn the skills to really reach your true potential and be willing to be in your fullness together. Play with any of the Embody It exercises in chapters seven to eleven.

It Comes Down to You . . .

I hope that you are leaving this chapter feeling hopeful about Blueprint pairings and excited to expand into new territory. And now you know your "mismatched" Blueprint pairing isn't doomed—in fact, it isn't a mismatch at all! Having different Blueprints mixed in one relationship can deepen creativity, open up options for exploration, and bring out some scintillating Superpowers.

Maybe you feel there are other issues holding you back from enjoying the sex you know you could be having. Not to worry, this is the perfect transition to our next chapter, where I'll introduce the ways you can become an Erotic Detective and share more about how you can expand your Erotic Blueprint. Learning how to problem-solve when challenges arise will help you transform your current obstacles into great sex and a lifetime of pleasure!

the four obstacles to sexual health and pleasure

There are four primary obstacles to sexual health and pleasure, and they can crop up at any time of your life. When left unchecked, they can become serious blocks to your sexual vitality and orgasmic potential.

For many of you, this may be the first time you've intentionally explored your sexual health and pleasure. This is understandable—sexuality support isn't always readily available or covered by health insurance. According to research, most doctors don't ask their patients about their sexual problems, sexual satisfaction, or pleasure. A 2018 survey found that only half of the medical schools in the United States required formal instruction in sexuality. No wonder so many of us are confused about sex.

The great news is, you can become your own Erotic Detective and transform these four Obstacles into pathways to optimal sexual health and pleasure.

Pleasure First: Celebrate!

So many of us never take the time to enjoy our successes, but celebrating our wins is important! Our brains are constantly looking to what is missing and what we haven't yet achieved. Celebration allows our brains to feel that we have grown and transformed, and to see that we have made strides in whatever our particular journey is. And celebrating is pleasurable!

Sit down with a journal, or do this exercise out loud with a lover. Light a candle or create a sacred space for celebration. You may even want to wear a party hat, if it brings you pleasure!

If you're doing this exercise with a partner, sit across from each other and take a moment to connect before you begin.

The prompt for this exercise is simply "Share something from your sexual journey that you want to celebrate."

Repeat this prompt to yourself or go back and forth with your partner for at least twenty minutes.

When the exercise is complete, treat yourself to a delicious dinner, read a good book, or get a massage. Do something to honor what you've achieved so far on your erotic journey.

Bonus points if you dine naked!

Obstacle #1: The Physical Realm

The Physical realm has to do with your body. This obstacle is anything physical that could stand in the way of great sex. For example, decreased range of motion in a joint, tight muscles, restricted blood flow. Anything that affects your nerves, muscles, joints, blood, and skin can create a sexual roadblock.

Let's take an inventory of your history to see what could be happening here.

» What surgeries have you had, and do you have any scar tissue from those surgeries?

» Do you suffer from any sort of chronic pain? If so, do you know the cause of that pain? What is that cause?

» Have you had any falls resulting in pelvic or spinal injuries? If so, how has this impacted your physical health and mobility?

» How is your flexibility? Do you have any mobility challenges?

» Do you have any chronic health problems such as a history of heart disease, respiratory illness, digestive disorders, thyroid disease, or any type of cancer? If so, how has this impacted your physical health and sex life?

» If you've had children, what was the birth like? Did you have an episiotomy, or do you have a C-section scar?

» Do you experience any pain during sex? If so, how does the pain prevent you from enjoying sex?

» Are you able to have and maintain erections?

» Do you have difficulty with premature ejaculation? If so, how is this preventing you from enjoying intimacy and sex?

» Are you able to have orgasms? If so, what is the quality of those orgasms?

These questions provide a starting point for thinking about anything in the Physical realm that could be holding you back from having the sex you seek.

Take a moment to write down whatever comes to mind. This is also the time to consider seeing a sex-positive coach and medical professional for help.

Pain often holds a person back from enjoying great sex. Unfortunately, painful intercourse is common, according to the American College of Obstetricians and Gynecologists. Almost three out of every four women experience pain during intercourse at some point in their lifetime. That's nearly 75 percent of all people with vaginas!

Erectile challenges (medically referred to as erectile dysfunction, or ED) are also incredibly common. An estimated 30 to 50 million men in the United States and 150 million men worldwide experience ED—and this is likely an underestimation, because many patients do not seek medical attention for ED, and many physicians are hesitant to inquire about their patients' sexual health. ED can be the result of taking certain prescription medication (which accounts for one-quarter of all ED cases), mental health issues, cardiovascular disease, or just normal aging.

Erectile challenges are also linked to an increased risk of cardiovascular disease. A meta-analysis of fourteen studies involving over ninety thousand men with ED revealed that they had 44 percent more cardiovascular events, 62 percent more heart attacks, 39 percent more strokes, and a 25 percent higher risk of death overall compared to patients who did not have ED. This means erectile dysfunction can be useful in predicting future cardiovascular events, which is why all ED patients should be screened for cardiovascular risk.

ED and challenges with premature ejaculation are so common that close to 90 percent of the men in my private practice over the past thirty years have been concerned about one or the other. It's a primary reason men come to see me—they want to last longer and be harder. But it's often not just a physical problem—it's commonly a combination of the four Obstacles, one of these being performance anxiety. Which links to the next realm—the Emotional.

Obstacle #2: The Emotional Realm

The Emotional realm is not as obvious as the Physical realm. A lot of challenges can lie in the subconscious areas of the mind, and even if we're conscious of past events that may have affected us, we don't connect those events to what is happening in our bodies now.

Any place where you currently have an emotional charge is a good place to start healing. Here's a list of questions to ask yourself to help you kick things off:

» What was your sex education like growing up? What hidden messages did you learn about sex? For example, did you learn that sex is shameful and taboo?

» What was your first experience of sex like? How did you feel afterward?

» What messages did you learn about relationships from your parents?

» What were your early relationships like?

» Did you experience any physical, emotional, or sexual abuse or trauma in your life? If so, how has that affected you?

» If you are in a relationship, how do you feel about that relationship and the person (or people) you are with? If you aren't currently in a relationship, how are you feeling about that?

» What experiences from your past have had the biggest influence on you?

» How do you feel about sex?

» How do you feel about your body? Do you like your body, or do you struggle with how you look? Why?

» Have you recently experienced any significant loss in your life, such as the death of a loved one? If so, how has that affected you?

» Are you feeling depressed or fearful, or struggling with a mental health challenge? If so, how does that affect your relationships?

I have found that the best processes for clearing emotional charges are those created by Serbian psychologist, teacher, and author Zivorad Slavinski. These processes, which Zivorad spent fifty years advancing, can relieve suffering and raise our emotional capabilities. Satyen Raja, founder of Warrior Sage, worked with Zivorad to create a methodology called Accelerated Evolution. Essentially, this methodology helps us clear strong emotional charges and brings us closer to having more compassion for ourselves and others.

Throughout this book, I have been giving you some of these processes, including the dyads on pages 54 and 55 and the prompted inquiries to the kenshō exercise on page 36. These processes should not be substituted for therapy, but can be used to relieve suffering caused by stuck emotions. Erotic Blueprint coaches have been trained in the Accelerated Evolution methodology and can help you transform emotions that are keeping you from pleasure.

It's also important to note that sometimes what seems like an emotional challenge is due to your biochemistry, part of the realm we'll explore next.

Obstacle #3: The Biochemical Realm

Have you had your hormones checked recently?

If not, it may be time to get a clearer picture of your Biochemical realm. The endocrine system is made up of several organs that secrete specific hormones, chemical messengers that tell your cells what to do. Many hormones impact your sexual health, which is why it's important to have these levels checked, especially as we age.

Basic blood work to check hormone and blood sugar levels could help you pinpoint a biochemical health issue that may be affecting your sexual function, which will enable you to seek out the right treatment plan for that issue. If you are going through menopause or andropause, this is especially important, because hormones play a big role in sexual health. Additionally, common conditions such as hypothyroidism are associated with decreased sex drive.

There are some other tests of your Biochemical realm available. These aren't standard in mainstream medicine, but I believe they may provide valuable insights into a person's individual biochemistry. A stool analysis, for example, can provide a breakdown of your gut microbiome, which is the ecosystem of beneficial and dangerous bacteria in your digestive system. This information can be significant, because research suggests a strong correlation between gut health and hormone levels.

If you want to dig deeper into the Biochemical realm of your health, you can seek out a functional medicine practitioner who is familiar with the range of less standard medical tests available to you. They can then order the tests for you, analyze the results when they come in, and help you understand what those results indicate.

Here are some questions to get you started in uncovering biochemical challenges:

» What prescription medications are you currently taking, and what is their effect on your sexual function?

» What supplements are you currently taking, and what is their effect on your sexual function?

» Are you partaking in any recreational drugs, and if so, what is their effect on your sexual function?

» Do you have a relationship with plant medicines, or are you taking part in psychedelic therapies? If so, what effect do those medicines have on your sexual function?

» How do mood swings affect you?

» Are you currently at the age of menopause or andropause? Are you on any supplemental hormone therapy? If so, how has the medication changed your interest in sex?

» Are you experiencing any spikes or crashes in your blood sugar? What are your symptoms?

» How is your gut health?

» Do you use any hormone disruptors, such as cleaning products, or have any in your home? If so, which ones?

My partner and I get blood tests at least once a year to find out what is happening in the Biochemical realm. This is how I discovered that my sex hormones had tanked after the birth of my son. After I gave birth, I felt very depressed, and came to find out that it wasn't as emotional as it was biochemical. Once I started bioidentical hormone therapy, I was back to myself again.

These yearly tests are also how I discovered that my mood swings were a result of blood sugar drops that happened just before my period would begin each month. It was so wonderful to find out the reason behind those anxiety-driven days and to work with my doctor to manage and treat the imbalances in a way that felt comfortable to me.

Frequently, when I'm working with clients with ED, we find from their blood work that they have low testosterone, something they might not even have considered. But after seeing their blood test results and working with their doctor to get their hormones in a healthy range, they have better success getting and maintaining erections.

It's always so rewarding when we can find easy solutions to what feel like insurmountable challenges. But sometimes, the mystery goes on, and that's when I look to the next realm.

Obstacle #4: The Energetic Realm

The Energetic realm is the trickiest and most misunderstood.

As humans, we are bioenergetic before we are physical or biochemical. Some research suggests that many common health disorders and diseases are at least partially energetic in nature, making them difficult to prevent or treat when not taken seriously in standard medical practices.

In this realm, we can uncover how our environment is affecting us at a cellular level, how energy flows through the body, and how our polarities, or energetic opposites, affect us.

Let's start with your environment.

» Are you aware of energy fields? If so, how sensitive are you to these fields? For example, when you hold your hand over your body, can you feel the energy?

» Do you have trouble falling asleep at night or get headaches from being on the computer for too long? If so, how does this interfere with your sex life?

» Can you feel electromagnetic fields (EMFs) around you? For example, if the TV isn't on, can you still sense a staticky feeling from it?

Each of us has energetic fields projecting from our bodies. As I mentioned in chapter seven, the effects of our field can be felt many feet away from our bodies by sensitive instruments designed to read these energetic fields.

The bioelectrical flows produced by organs such as the heart, brain, and muscles are the most well-documented energy fields. In clinical medicine, they are known by the technologies that measure them: the electrocardiogram, electroencephalogram, and electromyogram.

The energetic fields produced by the retina, nerves, lungs, ovaries, and other organs and glands are less well-known. In general, these energetic fields form due to the flow of electrical charges associated with virtually all physiological and regulatory processes in the body. Evidence shows that every event within the body is linked to measurable electrical activity.

So when your Energetic lover tells you they can feel you even when you're standing across the room, believe them.

Here are some questions to help you dig more deeply:

» Do areas of your body feel stuck and stagnant, but no one can find a physical or biochemical reason for that feeling?

» If you've ever had acupuncture, Reiki, or therapeutic touch treatments, can you feel them? Do they seem to work for you?

» Do you believe in the energy fields of the body and the principles of the ancient systems (Ayurveda, Chinese medicine, Indigenous healing wisdom) that first mapped them out?

» Can you feel subtle things happening in your body? If so, how would you describe these sensations?

And finally, we want to investigate polarities. Polarities are energetic opposites. With all my clients, we look at where these polarities attract, repulse, or fight against each other. I look at three main places that can have the greatest effect in a relationship:

» Masculine (yang) and feminine (yin) polarities (not to be confused with gender)

» Light (think angelic) and dark (think dangerous/Edgy) Polarities

» In Control or Surrendered

Here are some questions to get you started in examining how polarities are affecting you:

» Are you aware of polarized energies in your relationships or even within yourself? If so, how are these polarized energies affecting you?

» Do you feel you are more masculine energy or feminine energy? And is that where you would like to live? Where is your sweet spot?

» If you have a partner, do they feel the same about the polarity of masculine and feminine in you, or do they have a different view?

» When it comes to your sexuality, do you like to play more in light energy or dark energy? Do you feel that is your sweet spot, or would you like to change that?

» In the bedroom, are you more in control or more surrendered? Do you like where you are?

» Do you feel that the polarities you dance in are creating attraction or repulsion?

This book may be the first time you're reading about this. If you are interested in exploring more about polarities and how they relate to your erotic intelligence, you can seek out the help of an energy practitioner. Maybe start your own learning by getting a book on energy medicine or chakras.

Note: One thing to keep in mind as you are exploring these four Obstacles is that any sexual challenge can be a combination of some or all of these four realms. For example, a lack of arousal could be due to physical challenges related to blood flow; biochemical challenges from a medication you're taking; an emotional challenge that has arisen because you don't feel safe or connected to your lover; or a bioenergetic driver, where something is impeding the energy flow. Or all the above!

Accelerator and Brakes

The "accelerator and brakes" model was first popularized by Emily Nagoski in her book *Come As You Are*. The origin of that work was a theoretical model called the Dual Control Model of Sexual Response.

The Dual Control Model, developed in the late 1990s at the Kinsey Institute, is the current theoretical model of sexual response today. According to the Kinsey Institute, the Dual Control Model is based on the idea that sexual response in individuals results from "a balance between excitatory and inhibitory processes," which varies from person to person. The researchers compare it to a car having "both a gas pedal (excitation) and a brake pedal (inhibition)."

Each person engages one or both pedals in any sexual interaction, and this pattern of engagement is influenced by their physiology, personal history, and personality traits. I've come to realize that Blueprint Shadows and Obstacles are the brakes, while each Blueprint's individual turn-ons are the accelerator. Sexual risk-taking, infidelity, sexual aggression, sexual compulsivity, and even sexual satisfaction in couples have all been explained using the Dual Control Model.

No matter how much we put the accelerator on, if we have our foot on the brakes at the same time, we aren't going anywhere! And no matter how much we feed our Erotic Blueprint in all its turn-ons, we aren't going anywhere if we haven't healed the Shadows or transformed these four Obstacles into healthier territory.

Transform the Four Obstacles into Four Pathways for Optimal Sexual Health and Pleasure

When Noah came to me, he was unable to achieve an erection with a partner. He was fine during self-pleasure, but as soon as he was with a woman, he was unable to maintain an erection, and sometimes couldn't get one at all. He'd gotten to the point that he'd just given up on dating and having sex.

The last time Noah tried to have sex, he ended up having an anxiety attack, a profoundly embarrassing experience for him. After that, his therapist suggested he just stop trying for a while to lower the pressure.

This, however, didn't feel like a good solution to us. We had to look further...

When I start working with any new client, I do an intensive intake. We create their pleasure map by looking at their Sexuality Stage, Erotic Blueprint Type, and the Four Obstacles to Sexual Health and Pleasure.

Many men have shame about erectile function, and Noah was one of them. He hadn't talked to his doctor about medical issues that could be causing his challenge. And his doctor didn't ask.

"So, tell me about your physical body. How is your pelvic floor health? Have you had any surgeries? How is your flexibility? Any issues with circulation or heart health?" I peppered him with a few questions to help jar his memory about what might be going on with him physically.

"Well, I feel pretty good," he replied. "No heart issues that I know of. I did have reparative surgery about six months ago for a torn muscle, and they had to go through my groin. There's a thick scar on the left side," he revealed.

The buzzers in my head started to go off. Scar tissue can be a big issue when it comes to blood flow and function. I marked down in my notes that some scar tissue remediation or pelvic physical therapy work might be in order.

"Tell me about the last time you had your hormones checked," I continued. "How were your sex hormones?"

"I hadn't thought to get my hormones checked," he responded. "Do you think my testosterone might be low?"

I suggested that he talk to his doctor and have blood work done so that we could find out. Low testosterone, which falls under the biochemical Obstacle, could be a culprit.

Next we moved into the Emotional realm: "What happens when you go to have sex? What emotions do you feel? What thoughts are moving through your head, and how do those make you feel?"

"I feel like I can't win," he replied. "I feel like I can't do anything right. I just want to be confident when it comes to being with a lover, but I feel like a failure."

"It's hard to get hard when you feel like that," I told Noah. He nodded, clearly frustrated.

After going more deeply into his emotions and performance anxiety and feelings of panic, we eventually came to the Energetic realm. I started to ask him some questions to determine if he was sensitive to bioenergetic fields.

"Tell me, are you sensitive to EMFs or being on computer screens for long amounts of time? Are you aware of when a TV is plugged into the wall but not on, or sensitive to energy you feel in crowded places?" Then we went through some exercises to see if he could sense energy. From his response, we determined he didn't have much energetic sensitivity, but he did have some energetic polarities—namely, his masculine energy—that he wanted to improve. He wanted to feel more in charge and to have more of an edge as a lover, but he struggled, due to his inability to get and maintain an erection with a partner.

This is the process of being an Erotic Detective: Looking at all four Obstacles for possible challenges. Working with professionals in these areas can help you move through the Obstacles and transform them into optimized pathways for your pleasure.

We worked with Noah's doctor to get his blood tests (which showed that his testosterone was just fine).

I had him start working with Ellen Heed, a pioneer and expert in scar tissue remediation, education, and management (or STREAM). There was a lot of inflammation and thick scar tissue in his lower abdomen and groin that was transformed.

I helped him to clear all the emotional charges he had and addressed some of the misconceptions he had around erection, like thinking he had to be hard without any stimulation and remain hard for long amounts of time.

We gave him the skill sets he could use to calm his breathing and be able to pleasure a lover with his hands and mouth, taking the pressure off his penis.

And voilà! No issues with erection!

We used the four Obstacles to gain awareness of the issues at hand. And then we turned them into ways he could optimize his sexual health and pleasure. Noah could work with his team of doctors, me as his sexuality coach, his nutritionist, and his therapist to become his best possible erotic self and lover.

He started having sex again—his Primary Blueprint was Sexual—it made him so happy. He felt like he had his life back again.

This was not an overnight process. It took sleuthing, and it took some real courage for Noah to break through these obstacles.

The purpose of this chapter is to bring you more awareness and help you start asking useful questions to get to the bottom of any sexual challenges or Shadow aspects of your Blueprint.

With this Core Erotic Blueprint, you've been given an empowering map of sexual vitality that allows you to know who you are erotically, empowering you to claim the pleasure that is your birthright so you can more fully live in pleasure!

In the next chapter, I'm going to help you put this entire Erotic Blueprint Map together.

CHAPTER FIFTEEN

creating your core erotic blueprint map

If you were to place your pleasure journey on a map right now, where would you put yourself?

Deeply, orgasmically satisfied, and looking to fly to new heights?

Feeling some juicy goodness, but knowing there is more treasure to discover?

In the middle of the ocean? Or landlocked?

Lost and off course? Seeking signs to get you out of the dark forest and back on the pleasure path?

Or dying in the desert, praying to find an oasis?

Wherever you are on the map, it's best to recognize that *You Are Here!*

It's time to put some things together and create . . .

A map of your pleasure!

Pleasure First: Body Love

For this experience you will need either skin-safe paints and brushes or a skin-safe marker.

You may also want some fancy jewel stickers. Your body is the landscape, and the art supplies will help you create the map.

A pleasure map!

To start, stand naked in front of a mirror.

Write positive words, such as "I love you" or "Beautiful," all over your body. If you want, you can have a partner write words in places that are hard for you to see or reach yourself. Put sparkly sticky jewels all over yourself.

This is the artistry of self-love.

Place an X or a spiral on any of your hot spots, which you might have discovered during the body-mapping games in chapter twelve. Be creative and allow yourself to take your time creating the map.

This artistry is a way to integrate what you've learned about yourself, and if you have a lot of Sensual in your Blueprint, you may also enjoy the feeling of the markers or paintbrushes on your skin.

How can you make the creation of this map even more pleasurable?

As you look at your body and the work of art that your body and this map is, what delights your eyes?

To close, you may want to snap some creative pictures of certain places on your body. Photographs can be anchors that stop negative mind chatter and internal dialogues of body hating.

Journal about what you discovered as a result of doing this Pleasure First!

Your Core Erotic Blueprint Map

Your Core Erotic Blueprint consists of your Sexual Stage, your Erotic Blueprint Type, and the Four Obstacles to Sexual Health and Pleasure.

Putting these all together will help you awaken to where you currently are and allow you to design where you want to go next.

A little review before you put your Core Erotic Blueprint Map together . . .

THE FIVE STAGES OF SEXUALITY

- » Resting
- » Healing
- » Curious
- » Adventurous
- » Transformational

THE FIVE EROTIC BLUEPRINT TYPES

- » Energetic
- » Sensual
- » Sexual
- » Kinky
- » Shapeshifter

THE FOUR OBSTACLES TO SEXUAL HEALTH AND PLEASURE

- » Physical Realm
- » Emotional Realm
- » Biochemical Realm
- » Energetic Realm

When you look at your current sexuality as a blend of these three elements, you discover your Core Erotic Blueprint Map!

Here's my map as an example:

» I'm in the Adventurous and Transformational stages of my sexuality.

» I'm an Energetic Sexual.

» And my biggest Obstacles are currently in both the Physical and Biochemical realms.

After I had my son, my map was very different. I was in the Resting or Healing stage, and there was more emphasis on where the Obstacles were on my map and in healing those Obstacles. An Energetic who is Resting is a much different Energetic than one who is Curious or Adventurous.

The stage you're in matters. It also affects how you pair with a partner. My partner Ian is in the Adventurous stage of his sexuality, which works wonderfully when paired with my own adventurousness. He has expanded into a Kinky Sensual Shapeshifter. And his biggest Obstacles are currently in the Physical and Biochemical realms.

Knowing this about ourselves helps us navigate challenges when they come up, but it also helps us optimize our sexual health and pleasure for longevity and passion. We look like this:

Jaiya	Ian
Adventurous/Transformational	Adventurous
Energetic Sexual	Kinky Sensual Shapeshifter
Physical/Chemical	Physical/Chemical
Dryness	Low Libido
Estrogen Dominant	Low Testosterone
Pulling Sensation	Prostate Enlargement
Hypoglycemia with Period	Erectile Issues

This map is simply a product of your sexual history, what you learned early on in your sexuality journey, and the social conditioning you received from our sex-negative culture. Your map shows you the place from which you're starting.

Embody It: Create Your Map

Select three pages of your journal on which to do the following exercise.

Label the first page "My Sexuality Stage." In this section, write down the stage in which you currently find yourself and the stage you would like to be in. They may match, or they may not. Write down any feelings or discoveries you've made about your Sexuality Stage.

Now label the second page "My Erotic Blueprint Type." Write down your Primary and Secondary Erotic Blueprint Types. Then write down any important discoveries you made while doing body mapping or the A/B game (see pages 194 and 196).

Label the third page "My Four Obstacles to Sexual Health and Pleasure." Here you can write down the four realms and your obstacles. You may also want to write any action steps you want to take.

You don't necessarily have to write down words. Perhaps you want to draw pictures instead, or cut images out of magazines and tape them onto the page—like a mood board. You could also try finding poetry or quotes by other people that reflect how you feel about your map. Really take your time as you create your map, and be open to choosing new ways to express your thoughts. You may surprise yourself with what emerges on paper!

Take this one step further and share your map with a friend or lover. Discuss what you both discovered about yourselves in the process.

As you peel away these layers of conditioning and move into introspection, deep healing, and empowerment, you will discover something life-changing about yourself.

Your Sex Life Is a Game of Chess

Start thinking of your map as a chess game.

The board is the terrain upon which you're playing and is composed of factors such as the biochemistry of your body.

On that board are the players. You may be the queen or maybe you've thought of yourself as a pawn in your sexual journey. Whatever role you've played or others have played has shaped your game.

Finally, there are the rules of the game. The rules represent the conditioning and programming you've received throughout your life.

What happens when you make small adjustments to how the game is played? Or when you unravel the game completely, revealing all its secrets?

You discover that you can let go of the conditioning and roles you've been playing. You realize you can change the rules, even if those new rules seem unconventional and the game starts to not look like a game of chess at all! Suddenly, you've invented a new game entirely. How empowering! You become the designer of the game, instead of an unwitting player in a game you didn't realize you were stuck in.

And then . . . you are free!

Let me give you a more concrete example: Liz grew up in a very religious household. Her father was an alcoholic who literally beat the Bible into her. She was told from an early age to always be submissive to men and to a God that would punish her and send her to hell for eternity if she stepped out of line.

This was her programming.

Here are some of the rules to her game (her conditioning and programming):

» Good girls don't have sex.

» You will go to hell if you have sex before marriage.

» Just thinking about sex is wrong.

» You are a woman, and women should obey their fathers and their husbands.

» God is a punishing man who will send you to hell if you are not perfect.

» Sex is not about pleasure, it's for making babies.

» Birth control is wrong.

» Masturbation will definitely send you to hell.

» I'm bad and wrong for existing, so I deserve this abuse from others.

Here are some of the players on her board:

» Her father, who played the role of addict, abuser, punisher, and rule creator

» Her mother, who played the role of helpless victim and behaved how pious women should behave

» Her priest, who played the role of God's rule enforcer on earth.

» Her best friend, who played the role of rebellious, freely empowered woman

» Her therapist, who played the role of wise sage

» Herself, who played the role of Liz

And the terrain of her board:

» Liz was diagnosed with c-PTSD (complex post-traumatic stress disorder).

» Her ACE (adverse childhood experience) score was an 8 out of 10, which is very high.

» She struggled with feeling anxious and overwhelmed.

» She had never had an orgasm and had a very hard time having sex without feeling guilty, which affected her relationships.

» She was a Sensual Energetic Type with a lot of unhealed Shadow.

» She was in the Resting/Curious stage but wanted to be adventurous and free.

If Liz had passively accepted her circumstances, she might have gotten stuck in her trauma and her guilt about experiencing pleasure.

But Liz broke free.

How?

She courageously looked at her map and faced the present truth about it.

She became aware of things she hadn't seen before.

That was the first step. In looking at her terrain and all the people who played a role within it, and then looking at all the rules of the game that had been foisted upon her, she could see that the game she had played in her life was not who she really was.

This awareness was her first awakening.

She became so curious, she started to ask deeper questions.

What truly are my beliefs around sex? What are my beliefs about God? And what does God really have to say about sex? What were my parents teaching me that their parents taught them, and that just kept getting passed on generation by generation? What does science say about all of this? Was I really a monster just for existing?

As she began to question and get more introspective, she realized she was inviting new people in to be part of her game. She realized that she could choose a new board to play on as the terrain was changing. She realized she was choosing new rules that felt like they were true, ethical, and aligned with her own values, not those imposed upon her.

This process was her second awakening.

"I'm playing a new game here, and I get to choose it from my own lived experience and truth!" she told me as she started to design the game *she* wanted to play.

Embody It: Rewriting the Rules of Your Game

Get out your journal, some markers, magazines, and any other art supplies that you'd like to work with.

Make a list, cut images out of magazines, or draw pictures that you think represent the rules to your current sexuality game. Have fun with it and be creative.

If you're struggling, try filling in these blanks:

In my game, I'm expected to be _____.

People don't like it when _____.

I am not allowed to _____.

_____ is wrong.

Now glue in your pictures, draw, or make a list of all the players who have played vital roles in your game. Who influenced your sexuality, both positively and negatively? Who shaped your sense of self and made up the rules you had to follow in childhood and adulthood?

Take the next thirty to ninety minutes to rewrite the rules of your game. How do you want to play?

Use words, pictures, and art to reclaim your sexuality and create your own rules that feel like they empower you instead of subjugating you.

You may also include new players who you are inviting to play with you in the future. Maybe this is a skilled lover. Or perhaps a mentor who can guide you to where you want to go. Or you may even consider a sex-positive group you want to get involved with.

And then Liz began some of the deepest work on this journey. The third step of sexual awakening.

Who am I?

In deeply asking this question, she realized that even her identity was unfixed. She was malleable.

She didn't need to defend any part of herself.

She was free to choose her form. Free to choose her identity.

She could play the angel or the whore. She could be the sweet shy girl, or she could be the Dominant persona who took complete control.

She was free to play with any identity she desired. In fact, she was all identities and no identities at all.

Now she was off the board.

Now she could play any role at any time. She could choose any game she wanted to play. Now, instead of asking who she was, she could ask what kind of experience she wanted to have.

How fun is that?

This was yet another awakening for Liz, and just the beginning of her adventure toward living a fully expressed life as her truly found self.

Once, Twice, Three Times a Sexual Awakening

From what I have seen in my practice and from my own personal experiences, multiple awakenings can happen on this journey.

FIRST SEXUAL AWAKENING—QUESTIONING YOUR REALITY: At first you can't see the game you are playing, but you keep asking questions and peeling away the layers and layers of conditioning and programming. You question what you are programmed to think. You question who and what you are. You begin to realize you don't know what you don't know. Until you do. And then you wake up to the game you've been playing.

SECOND AWAKENING—CREATING YOUR REALITY: You now fully see the game you've been playing, and you begin to reclaim and rewrite the rules of that game. You start to get a taste of freedom. You begin to have glimpses of who you are as an erotic being and start to live by what you know to be true, without the influence of past conditioning and programming. You truly begin to love and accept yourself.

THIRD SEXUAL AWAKENING—TRUTH: You discover deeper truths about yourself and this cosmic game. You are no longer playing unless by choice; you can leave the board and the game behind, because there's no need for you to play anymore. You realize that you are *you*. But, also, that your identity isn't fixed. It's malleable. You see you are magnificent and extraordinary.

If you are reading these words, then I trust that one day you are going to have this awakening.

But here's the trick, the riddle: There is no place to get to.

You're already here.

Your Blueprint Type shows you a current truth about your sexuality. But this current expression of who you are reveals where you've limited yourself. And it shows that you haven't developed or allowed yourself to move beyond that identity and develop into the other Blueprint Types. (I'll go further into how you can expand and explore the different Blueprint Types in the next chapter.)

I have a theory. It comes from years of watching people on this journey of sexual awakening and coming into the truth of who they really are.

My theory is that we are all Shapeshifters.

It's just that our sexual richness and full expression gets shamed, conditioned, and programmed out of us. We learn what's safe and acceptable, and then we create a reality based on that. We have certain life experiences or traumas, and then we learn to defend the identities we create based on those life experiences.

Slowly, our big sexual natures get put into little boxes, and then we wonder why we feel dull and unfulfilled—even when our circumstances of life look pretty good.

There Is a Place Beyond the Blueprints

There is a place where you rest in the richness of who you are, free to be you, in peak existence...

This entire book has been an invitation into that place.

I'll meet you there.

Or, in the famous words of the Sufi poet Rumi:

Out beyond ideas of wrongdoing and rightdoing,

There is a field. I'll meet you there.

When the soul lies down in that grass,

The world is too full to talk about.

Ideas, language, even the phrase each other

Doesn't make any sense.

Have I sparked your curiosity? Made you wonder how you can start to play a different game? Now that you have the tools to make a map of your pleasure, you have a choice to make.

Will you continue to play the same game that you are playing and keep getting the same results?

Will you choose the next, courageous step on the path? The step of conscious awakening?

Or will you keep doing what you've been doing and expecting different results (which is the definition of insanity, by the way)?

I ask you these questions with great love. What will you choose?

CHAPTER SIXTEEN

feeding, speaking, healing, and expanding your erotic blueprint

Laughter in big bellows sounded through the room. You could feel the ecstasy thick in the air.

His back arched, his spine waved in deep, unfolding undulations.

We were eight hours into his immersion with his lover. For the past three hours, we'd been breathing and touching and feeding him in his Shapeshifter Blueprint. A year ago, he'd been starving, stuck in a longing and a craving that was painful for him. The pain turned to anger. He was considering leaving his relationship because he knew there was something more for him, and he yearned to experience it.

His lover looked at me with a twinkle in her eyes.

"Deep breath in. Breathe up your spine. Hold it. Hold it. Squeeze your whole body," I instructed, giving him some reminders of techniques for transmuting sexual energy that he'd learned during his one-year journey of learning from me.

"Exhale when you are ready."

He squeezed and held and then let out a big release. And then . . .

He laughed and laughed.

All the unexpressed joy he'd held inside his entire life came spilling out.

His partner began laughing, too, and I couldn't help but catch the bug myself. His laughter was contagious.

"I am joy!" he exclaimed.

"Have you always been this joy?" I asked him.

Another bellow of laughter rocked his body. "Yes, yes! I'm *me!*" And now he wept and laughed and shook all at once.

Then he sat bolt upright. He looked his lover straight in her eyes.

"I'm me! It's all so perfect. All of it . . . led to this. Love."

They held each other. And they wept together.

A tear trickled down my own cheek.

After what seemed like a timeless moment, he looked over at me and asked, "Now what?!?"

"Now you play," I replied. "Now begins a new journey. Now you know who you truly are, so now you *live* like you know."

He took a deep breath. We wrapped him in blankets and fed him some sweet fruits, and his partner drew a luxurious bath for them to dip into together.

Ah, the sweetness of remembering our true essence.

By now you have a pretty good understanding of who you've been conditioned to be. You're beginning to get closer to who you truly are as an erotic being. Remembering who you are doesn't always come with the phenomenon of ecstasy like the experience you just read about.

Sometimes it's quiet. A simple realization.

Sometimes it's in tears. A surrendering and letting go into truth.

The phenomenon and the way it occurs are not important. What *is* important is the direct experience of uncovering a truth about yourself.

Once you know your map, you can begin this next leg of the journey. After that, it's time to adventure and to play in a different way—which requires you to create a new map.

There are four next steps, which I'll lay out in a moment. These steps have many benefits, which we'll explore here. But before we do, you have a choice to make.

Are you willing to take the next step? Are you ready to put your new map to use and eventually put the map/game down and play in a way that may feel completely foreign to you? If you're in a relationship, are you ready to innovate, to let go of the memories of the past and the imaginings of the future and create a new relationship here and now?

If the answer is yes, then let's dive in further together.

If it's maybe or no, it might be good to revisit your first map and see where your resistances lie. If you're a hard no, it might be time to accept where you are in your sexuality right now. I'm going to remind you again that you are whole and complete just the way you are. Nothing is broken. But if you are in a relationship, your self-acceptance may mean changes in your relationship so that your partner can also have their needs met.

Quickie Pleasure First: The Ordinary Extraordinary

Breathe in. Breathe out.

Notice the simple pleasure of your breath.

It's that easy.

Four Action Steps

ACTION #1: FEEDING

When it comes to feeling satisfied sexually, most people don't.

Being fed is a practice of satiation, especially for Shapeshifters.

Being fed means that you feel full erotically, you feel satisfied with plea-sure, and from this full cup of love you can feed others, without feeling resentful or depleting yourself.

Being fed means that you can feed yourself in your Blueprint and that you are able to receive from and give pleasure to your lover in a skillful, loving way. You can confidently satisfy your lover's desires and honor their Primary Blueprint, even if it differs from your own.

When you are fed, you have the capacity to spill over with generosity.

Just like food, if we are starving, we have low energy, we are focused on ending the discomfort of hunger. But when we eat, we feel better. If we eat food we love, food that is nutritious and high quality, and it is available to us without fear of it being taken away, then we can feel satiated.

BLUEPRINTIFYING SEX TIPS

Getting creative with techniques and feeling comfortable and confident enough to explore new territory is a challenge for many people, and can stop them from taking control of their journey. A great way to find tech-niques to feed you in the bedroom and build your confidence is to take any technique and Blueprintify it.

What do I mean by that?

Well, you simply take a technique—from any book on sex or any magazine that shares sex tips—then identify which Blueprint that technique belongs to by the way the technique is described. (HINT: Almost *all* sex techniques offered in popular media are geared toward the Sexual Blueprint.)

Embody It: Simple Feeding Experience

Set aside some time to get fed. This can be a short session of fifteen minutes, just to give you a taste and a quick win.

Here are some ideas for each Blueprint:

ENERGETIC: Hover your hands over your body and then give yourself light energetic fingertip touch from head to toe.

SENSUAL: Massage yourself with scented oils you find pleasing.

SEXUAL: Touch your genitals with various strokes that feel good.

KINKY: Give yourself some intense sensation, such as scratch or slap.

SHAPESHIFTER: Try everything above and in different combinations.

After your practice, make notes of what you'd like more of, what didn't work for you, and what you'd like to try with a lover.

The final step is to rework it to appeal to all the Blueprint Types.

Here's an example:

Original Technique: Ring Fingers for Blueprintified Blow Jobs

Take your thumb and forefinger and form the shape of an O. Wrap this ring around the penis at the base and pull the skin taut to expose more nerve endings. Now suck the head of the penis.

Obviously, this is a Sexual technique.

Let's Blueprintify it!

Energetic

Take your thumb and forefinger and form the shape of an O.

Very slowly, while looking into your lover's eyes, take this ring and glide it down their erect penis without touching, or barely touching, their skin.

Stop at the base of their penis and hold. Now use your breath on the head of their penis, then put the head barely in your mouth without touching it with your lips, tongue, or teeth.

Sensual

Make sure to use some coconut oil or other delicious-tasting oil for this technique.

Take your thumb and forefinger and form the shape of an O. Gently and with firm pressure glide this ring from the head of their penis down to the base. Do this a few times while your other hand rubs their inner thighs or chest.

Now slowly lick between their thighs and their genitals, working your way to their penis, which you can lick with long strokes.

Sexual

Stays the same as originally described above!

Take your thumb and forefinger and form the shape of an O.

Wrap this around their penis at the base and pull the skin taut to expose more nerve endings. Now go to town, sucking the head.

Kinky

If you're in a more Dominant role, tell them they aren't allowed to squirm, make a sound, or orgasm until you say so. (If you're in a more service-oriented role, come in service and submit to their pleasure.)

Now take your thumb and forefinger and form the shape of an O.

Slowly pull this ring down from the head of their penis to the base; this will expose more nerve endings.

With your other hand and your mouth, you can tease them with pleasure. If they squirm or squeal and you've instructed them not to, stop and give them the agreed-upon punishment for their disobedience.

They get to orgasm only if you say so.

Shapeshifter

Start by looking into your lover's eyes. Take a few deep breaths together.

Now massage with oil from their heart to their genitals and down their thighs.

Now take your thumb and forefinger and form the shape of an O. Wrap this ring around their penis at the base and pull the skin taut to expose more nerve endings.

Now suck the head of their penis.

Tell them they are not allowed to orgasm until you say so. Go to town, teasing and pleasuring them but controlling their orgasm.

If you are not the one in control (the Dominant in this scenario), you can act in service, looking into your lover's eyes and asking them to tell you exactly what to do.

Now it's your turn.

Choose any of your favorite sex tips and Blueprintify them!

ACTION #2: SPEAKING THE BLUEPRINTS

When we talk about "speaking" the Blueprints, we're talking about your body language and the tone of voice you use to communicate. Communication is so much more than our words. We are reading body language, facial expression, and vocal tone.

My Energetic lover says that we vibrate each other with our voices. When he speaks, it's like he's making love to me; the words he's using don't matter so much.

I find this so sexy.

How are you being vibrated by your amour? How are you vibrating your lover? Does your lover believe you when you speak, or gesture with your body?

I hear this common complaint a lot in my practice and in working with coaches: "I just don't feel like I'm seen or understood."

Imagine a world where we've all learned this art of helping each other feel deeply seen, deeply heard, and deeply understood. This is the essence of a truly loving relationship: Seeing love as an active verb and not something passive that happens to us. Actively being this loving presence, in service to ourselves and others, is the cherished art of love and passion, and it's something we have largely forgotten how to do.

Speaking your lover's Blueprint means loving them by learning the words they love to hear and speaking those words exactly when they love to hear them. Saying these words in a vocal tone and with body language that matches the energy behind them is mastery. This is especially true for Energetic and Kinky Types who are going to pick up on all the subtle vibrations. Both these types can sniff out incongruence and lack of alignment in a second, and that creates a complete disconnect from surrendering to pleasure.

This is not to say that you want to overthink all of this. If you're overthinking it, you aren't in it. It simply takes practice and getting comfortable adapting your identity to play in different Blueprint styles—to shapeshift yourself!

Embody It: Quickie Aural Sex Game

You will need a partner to read a list of words to you.

While they are reading the words, feel the level of arousal in your body. When they're done reading, report which words turned you on the most.

» **WORDS FOR GENITALS:** Pussy, Slit, Hot Pocket, Cunt, Portal
» **WORDS FOR GENITALS:** Cock, Dick, Vajra, Wand, Meat Stick
» **WORDS FOR SEX:** Fucking, Making Love, Becoming One, Having Sex, Banging
» **WORDS FOR BEDROOM:** Tantric Temple, Fuck Room, Sanctuary of Delights, Boudoir, Dungeon

This is a great start to see what kinds of words work well in the heat of the moment. You can also try playing this game with a lover and experimenting with different vocal tones and body language.

Make a note of what turns you on the most, and be sure to communicate this to your lover so you can try out these words when you are making love or fucking or whatever word you like best for "banging"!

ACTION #3: HEALING THE BLUEPRINT

Healing is one of the most empowering steps you can take when it comes to creating a different and rewarding map for your pleasure.

This is where you want to look at the Shadow aspects of your Blueprint(s) and the Four Obstacles to Sexual Health and Pleasure. Healing means taking the Shadow aspects and Obstacles that are putting the brakes on your pleasure and unwinding their grip.

Healing is about integrating those aspects so they're no longer driving the bus. They no longer have control. You do.

You can turn all Obstacles into pathways to optimal pleasure and health.

How do we know that healing has occurred?

The negative pattern or block no longer shows up. It's completely gone. Or perhaps the pattern shows up, but it no longer bothers you. For example, in the past you found it very distressing that your partner isn't as interested in sex as you are, but now it doesn't matter like it used to.

Or maybe the pattern shows up, but in a different way! For example, in the past, your partner wasn't interested in sex, but now they are, and now *you* are distressed because they don't want to spend as much time hiking with you as they used to.

Healing means that you've changed the terrain; that the old and corrupted map has been replaced by a treasure map of possibilities.

Healing is powerful and empowering.

You do not, however, want to constantly chase healing.

There is a place in each of us where we have healed enough.

There is a time and a place where radical self-acceptance and unconditional love are the appropriate practice.

Let Sex Be Your Medicine!

Sexual health is a vital yet often overlooked part of overall well-being. Numerous studies link sex with better physical and mental health. Healing and connecting with aspects of your sexuality make it possible for you to reap the benefits of good sexual health and vitality.

Here are just a few of the benefits related to sex that you may be unaware of:

» Relaxation and calming: Sex can feel relaxing because sexual arousal lowers levels of cortisol, a stress hormone. Lower cortisol levels can help reduce anxiety and chronic stress over time.

» Boost immune function: Sex significantly raises your levels of immunoglobulin A (IgA), an important antibody that is part of your immune system.

» Better aging: One study found that feelings of well-being are higher among older adults who are sexually active.

» Better sleep: Orgasm increases levels of prolactin and oxytocin, hormones that help promote sleep and relaxation, so having sex may make it easier to fall asleep.

ACTION #4: EXPANDING YOUR BLUEPRINTS

Expanding is the ability to have access to the turn-ons of other Blueprints. Expanding can look like trying new sexual dynamics that are outside any conditioning or programming you experienced previously in your life.

When you expand, you become a more masterful lover. If you continue expanding, you'll eventually become a fully-developed Shapeshifter in your giving, which means you can please any of the Erotic Blueprint Types.

In other words, you can become the ultimate lover!

Expanding means liberating yourself from any limiting beliefs and starting to experience the magnificent erotic being you truly are! It allows you to awaken to and explore more of the fullness of *you*. Expanding has you in the driver's seat, creating the game, the players, and the rules by which you play!

You become an infinite erotic creation and creator all in one!

And then there is no end to the infinite pleasure possibilities that await you.

These four action steps are the key to taking everything you've learned here to the next level. I could fill books with ways to accomplish this, which is why learning these arts is a lifetime journey.

At some point, your erotic creativity becomes so natural that you no longer have to think about how to *do* it—it just comes authentically from who you are.

It's a truly beautiful thing.

As we bring this journey to a close, I want to share with you one more framework to help you create hot sex for the rest of your *life*!

If you haven't guessed, this is an invitation into a new game, a new paradigm, a new life, even a new world, in which all of us can live free of shame and full of pleasure . . .

Embody It: Creating an Empowered Erotic Persona

Personas can help you to integrate Shadow aspects and expand into exciting and unfamiliar places.

Reclaim your eroticism that has been lost, buried, shamed, or hidden.

For example, my Erotic Persona, whose name is Puddles, allowed me to reclaim the very sexual aspect of myself that is innocent and filled with delight for life!

Because I had been shamed for my sexual nature throughout my life, I had lost my ability to be unabashedly, overly sexual.

Puddles has no issue being overtly sexual and bursting with delight.

Erotic Personas are not role-playing; rather, they are deep, authentic aspects of ourselves that we have buried or disowned and are bringing back to light.

The first step is to choose what you would like to reclaim. Whatever you choose to expand into needs to feel like an easy win for you; otherwise, the exercise may overwhelm you.

Ask yourself:

What Erotic Blueprint Type is this persona?
What am I reclaiming about my sexuality?
Who would I be if I fully stepped into this persona?

How does this persona act in the bedroom?
How do they like to be erotically fed?
How do they dress?
What do they most desire?
What does their voice sound like?
How does this persona move?

Make a drawing or create a vision board for this persona.
Spend a few hours playing as this persona.

Dress as this persona. Self-pleasure as this persona, or
make love to your partner as this persona. (If your partner is
involved, warn them of what you're doing beforehand—I've had
more than one client report that their lover freaked out when
someone new showed up in their bed unannounced.)

I take six weeks to develop each persona of my own and
when working with clients, and this development period
culminates with a photo shoot. It helps to integrate the persona
more fully, and it's so much fun to see yourself completely
transformed through the magic of photography.

CHAPTER SEVENTEEN

creating hot sex for a lifetime

Congratulations!

You've made it through an extraordinary journey that has brought you more awareness and experiences of your erotic self!

At this point in the journey, you may be wondering what's next. I would like to leave you with one final framework to contemplate and put into action in your life.

Know Your Pleasure, Own Your Pleasure, Live Your Pleasure

Deep love and unbridled, lasting passion are goals for so many couples.

Most of my clients want it all—inside *and* outside the bedroom.

What most of them don't understand when they step onto the path of sexual awakening is that pleasure is a lifelong journey. They want sexual mastery but don't realize that sexual mastery means being aware that you never stop learning about sex and about yourself.

Pleasure First: Experiencing the Music

Part of creating hot sex for a lifetime is having the ability to experience the moment fully. One way that we teach practicing this is with music.

Challenge: Can you experience a song, in pleasure, from start to finish?

Put your sexiest favorite song on and truly experience the song in the most pleasurable way possible, staying present with each delicious note.

What way of staying present in the music feels best and most comfortable for you?

Is it singing along with your full voice?

Is it dancing for joy in celebration of this erotic journey?

Is it making love to yourself, your hands gliding deliciously across your skin?

Is it lying in a pile of pillows and feeling the sound wash over you?

Is it rolling around in your bed naked as the notes dance in your bones?

Is it making love with a partner or just lying next to each other while listening to the song?

Allow yourself to block out all the interruptions of life and take time to indulge in the music! If you notice yourself drifting, start the song over. This exercise is complete only when you have been fully present, experiencing the song, from start to finish.

The conclusion of this book is not the end of your journey—it's just the beginning. So how do you explore and expand into erotic possibilities for the rest of your life?

There are three phases, and you've already begun . . .

PHASE ONE: KNOWING YOUR PLEASURE

After reading this book, I'm certain you are well on your way to knowing your pleasure.

Knowing your pleasure means you've uncovered your Sexuality Stage, you've determined your Erotic Blueprint Type, and you know what's standing in your way with the Four Obstacles to Sexual Health and Pleasure. You have come to know yourself better and perhaps you're now better able to communicate your needs and desires with a partner. Knowing your pleasure also means you realize that none of these elements is fixed. You are able to choose who you are as an erotic being and are now ready for the next step.

Knowing your pleasure is also about learning the skill sets for both pleasing a partner and feeding yourself. What could you learn today to enhance your skills as a lover?

PHASE TWO: OWNING YOUR PLEASURE

Owning your pleasure is accepting where you àre now and fully owning it!

It's about claiming your bodily autonomy and saying what you want and don't want. This is the phase where you can now feed, speak, heal, and expand your Blueprints with ease.

You can put all you've learned into practice.

PHASE THREE: LIVING YOUR PLEASURE

Living your pleasure is when your work in the erotic world is fully integrated into your life.

You may have realized a phase three sexual awakening and live from the truth of who and what you are. You are no longer needing to practice; you realize that you are pleasure, and you generate the pleasure you crave. Pleasure is no longer something that you seek to receive—pleasure is who you are.

Loving Yourself Through It All

At the core of these three phases is a process of learning to love yourself more fully. It is not cliché to love yourself, because when you love yourself, everything changes.

You make healthy boundaries, you have consent conversations, you only have sex that you truly want to have, and you can love others in a way that leaves them free to be fully who they are.

I come back to this phrase that a dear mentor once shared with me: *Unconditional love for you, from you, then everyone gets it.*

The day I truly realized and felt this truth, all my relationships transformed overnight. Yours will, too.

My sexual life became so ease-filled, because there was nothing more that I needed to do, be, or have in order to be loved.

When you realize this, you will no longer seek love and pleasure from outside yourself, and you will be full of love and pleasure in all ways.

And love yourself through it all. Unconditionally.

Yes, I know that can be easier said than done. It's so simple, and yet such a profound daily practice.

All the pleasure you seek is right here, right now, in you.

I also want to give you some concrete suggestions that my lover Ian and I do to continue to deepen our intimacy, expand our love, and cultivate hot sex for the rest of our lives.

HIRE MENTORS, COACHES, AND GUIDES: Ian and I have always had someone there to support us. We've worked with a ton of mentors, coaches, and guides to address sexual health issues, work through unresolved trauma, and help us remember who we really are. When hiring mentors, it's important that you feel confident that they can help you and are in alignment with your needs. Make sure you hire people who lead you back to yourself, your truth. You do not want to work with people who make the experience about how they are the solution to challenges you are facing.

Hire someone who is both skilled and compassionate and who has had their own sexual awakenings. I'd also recommend finding someone with a somatic background, because sexual awakening happens not just in your head, but in your body as well. It's also critical that you make sure the coach or mentor you hire has a great reputation for ethical practices, understands and practices consent, and honors boundaries. Inquire about what code of ethics they follow and what consent guidelines they currently practice from. Ask about their credentials and who served as their own mentors.

See page 287 for a list of resources to help you get started with your search for the right coach or mentor.

PRACTICE WHAT YOU PREACH: If you just stay in the world of concepts and do not put things into practice, you are not building skill and mastery. We regularly practice what you read in this book. We do the Embody It exercises, we have Pleasure First as a core life value, we play with Erotic Personas, we do sex life practices, we make love feeding each other's

Blueprints. Sometimes we do need a coach to help hold us accountable to our practices or to teach us new skills when neither of us has those skills, or if we've forgotten, for a moment, who we are.

For example, I might hire a kink expert to help us put into practice feeding Ian's Kinky Blueprint in ways that I don't know how.

What can you put into practice?

We can all find time to practice something erotically. Even if it's only fifteen minutes a week. How can you weave what you've discovered in this book into your life? In what ways can you, as one of my mentors, Wesly Feuquay, phrased it, "live like you know"? What kind of support do you need to make that happen?

THE POWER OF EROTIC COMMUNITY: Being part of a community that is working together toward sexual freedom can really enlighten your mind. It's another way of having support, especially if the community is cultivated to have consent conversations, to love themselves, and to be freer in their erotic expression.

I've been part of many erotic communities along my path, and I've suffered from boundary breaks and unethical behavior in many of those communities. It's tragic that people seeking a safer place to explore their vulnerable and sensitive side are often harmed or retraumatized in erotic communities where consent is not practiced and there is no ethical standard being practiced to help create safety.

In our search for an erotic community to join, Ian and I didn't find any that we felt safe in to explore *all* aspects of our sexuality, so we created our own inclusive community, Erotic Freedom Club, based on the values of consent, freedom, and inclusivity.

We wanted a place where all Blueprints, all orientations and relationship styles were welcome—a place where everyone could feel safe, and could feel free to be who they truly are.

One of the biggest challenges we've seen our clients face in trying to find solutions to their sex life challenges is isolation. If you haven't noticed, there aren't many quality resources out there in the world to help you learn about sex and pleasure. Pursuing a path of pleasure, speaking openly and honestly about it, is shamed in our culture. You reading this book is, in fact, a radical act.

Continuing to struggle in isolation, trying to figure it out all alone and on your own, is often a recipe for failure. Finding a community of support, or creating your own, can support you on your sometimes challenging journey of erotic awakening. When you hit a roadblock, there are people to help you break through. When you have a breakthrough, there are people to cheer you on and celebrate your wins.

I've provided some resources to help you connect with like-minded people on page 288.

My Prayer for You Is This

As a result of reading this book, you see your full magnificence and love yourself deeper than ever before.

I envision for you a life fully expressed, filled with pleasures that you've never imagined possible.

I imagine a world where you are so embodied and empowered and in love with yourself that your radiance spills over into everyone you meet.

I envision that your Being is so contagious, it inspires others into their own journeys of awakening.

Can you see it too?

What a wonderful world we can create together.

I see a world where this book and the conversation about the Erotic Blueprints opens people to more play and more passion, deeper connection, and unconditional love.

Embody It: Integration

The point of exploration is to discover new things and bring those discoveries and wisdoms back with you. These are your seeds.

Go to your journal and write down the following:

What are the discoveries I have brought back with me?
What do these things mean to me?
How will I nurture these seeds?

Here's an example:

Seeds I'm bringing back

» I can explore my sexuality free of shame.
  • I will do one thing each week to express my new freedom.
» I'm a Shapeshifter, which means I love it all and want it all.
» I will nurture this seed by exploring all the Erotic Blueprints, and will find other Shapeshifters to explore with.

Don't stomp on your new growth if the transformation isn't bearing fruit quickly enough. Revisit this list each week to make sure you are nurturing the seeds you've brought back with you.

You will know you've fully integrated this new growth when the extraordinary experiences feel ordinary, and you are operating from a new baseline in your life.

I believe that pleasure can bring the world to a peaceful place, and I hope that as you come to the end of this writing, you too see how pleasure changes your world and the relationships around you.

How you, living in pleasure, ripple out to transform the entire world.

Be you.

Be love.

And let's inspire others to do the same.

Until next time . . .

Fill your heart with love and your life with pleasure,

Jaiya

acknowledgments

From conception to creation, the book you are holding in your hands has been over a decade-long labor of love. Birthing a book is no easy feat. It takes a team of people to make it all happen.

First and foremost, there is a man in my life who has not only adventured alongside me as my life partner, but who supports me unconditionally. He has taken the Erotic Blueprints and helped me create a brand and a legacy. He is often the one to test out all the exercises and sexual antics I come up with. My beloved Ian Ferguson, thank you so much for everything you are and everything you do for this dharma.

The "Angelas," who are amazing supporters and powerhouse women: Angela Thurston, thank you for your attention to detail, for loving this mission, for being by Ian's side, and for everything you contribute creatively to the Erotic Blueprint brand. Angela Ruggiero, whew, thank you for creating the space for me to finally be able to write this book. What has it been, five years? Thank you for being so willing to manage all the people and the projects so that Ian and I can bring our brilliance!

Marti Stany, wow, woman! You are a force of good for the world. Thank you for your wonderful mind and work ethic. Thank you for helping me with all the research for this book, which made it a more enriching learning experience for every reader.

Thank you to Linda Loewenthal, my literary agent, who has for years supported me as a writer and educator. Thank you for all the books you've helped bring into the world and all the writers whose voices you believe in. Thank you for believing in me during this whole process (even when I wanted to throw in the towel)!

Thank you to Jessica Firger and the team at Union Square for all the editorial work on this project—you made this book more relatable and accessible to readers.

acknowledgments

Thank you to Amy Stanton, Dana Lewis, and the Stanton and Co. team who launched this book into the world through their amazing work in publicity! It's so delightful to work with people who are behind a sex-positive voice in the world. Thank you for believing in us.

To all my clients: You are so brave. I am in awe of your courage, and of your transformations. I'm grateful and honored each day to be able to do this work in the world. It's because of you that this book is rich with stories in which readers can find themselves. Thank you.

All of our Erotic Blueprint coaches, wow, we have been on such a journey together! Lead Trainers, I'm so grateful that the Erotic Blueprint Methodology will live on beyond my days. Lea Newman, Anne More, Connie Eberhart, Genevieve, and Angela Thurston, thank you for being the originals!

My family, both by blood and by soul, and my lovers, thank you all for understanding my time away to write this book. Thank you for being so supportive and for being there for me in all ways. Jon Hanauer, Christian Duhamel, and Michael Ashley, thank you for loving me and doing all the things to keep me resourced in pleasure. I love you all. I'm so grateful for your willingness to have our stories shared, to be an example of love for the world.

And finally, to my mentors: Joseph Kramer, Kenneth Ray Stubbs, Bodhi Avinasha, Carista Luminare, Jack Morin, Esther Perel, Ellen Heed, Satyen Raja, Wesly Feuquay, and Doc: Without you, this book and this methodology would not be possible.

resources for sexual health, awakening, and discovery

Core Erotic Blueprint Resources

THE IN-DEPTH EROTIC BLUEPRINT QUIZ/ASSESSMENT
theblueprintbreakthrough.com
The Blueprint quiz reveals your Primary Erotic Blueprint Type. The in-depth assessment details your complete "Pleasure Profile," which shows you how you uniquely relate to sex through each of the five Erotic Blueprint Types. This personalized pleasure map shows you the many routes to creating a life filled with healthy intimacy, sexy vitality, and sexual satisfaction.

THE EROTIC BLUEPRINT BREAKTHROUGH COURSE
theblueprintbreakthrough.com/ebbc
This is our flagship Erotic Blueprint Training. It's an eight-module online course providing a comprehensive exploration and expansion of the Erotic Blueprints.

ALL COURSES AVAILABLE FROM THE BLUEPRINT BREAKTHROUGH, INC.
missjaiya.com/program
This is where you can access all our currently available courses, live workshops, luxury retreats, and trainings.

THE EROTIC BLUEPRINT COACH DIRECTORY
missjaiya.com/coach-directory
Find a Certified Erotic Blueprint Coach for personalized support. Please note that Blueprint Coaches are independent contractors and operate independently of the

Blueprint Breakthrough, Inc. A Blueprint Coach is required to adhere to set ethical standards to retain their certification.

SEX-POSITIVE ONLINE COMMUNITY—EROTIC FREEDOM CLUB
eroticfreedomclub.com
This is our membership community, where the Erotic Blueprints are the foundational framework. We offer trainings, group coaching support, and a safer space to explore all that is erotically possible.

Blueprint-Related Products and Toys

theblueprintbreakthrough.com/products
This is a list of our current recommended pleasure-enhancing toys and products organized by Blueprint Type.

Further Reading

Cuffed, Tied, and Satisfied: A Kinky Guide to the Best Sex Ever by Jaiya (Harmony, 2014)

Blow Each Other Away: A Couples' Guide to Sensational Oral Sex by Jaiya (Harmony, 2013)

Red Hot Touch: A Head-to-Toe Handbook for Mind-Blowing Orgasms by Jaiya and Jon Hanauer (Harmony, 2008)

The Erotic Mind: Unlocking the Inner Sources of Passion and Fulfillment by Jack Morin, PhD (Harper Perennial, 1996)

Jewel in the Lotus/The Tantric Path to Higher Consciousness by Bodhi Avinasha (Ipsalu Publishing, 2002)

Mating in Captivity: Unlocking Erotic Intelligence by Esther Perel (Harper Paperbacks—Reprint, 2017)

Holotropic Breathwork: A New Approach to Self-Exploration and Therapy by Stanislav Grof, MD, and Christina Grof (Excelsior Editions 2010)

The Way of the Psychonaut: Encyclopedia for Inner Journeys by Stanislav Grof, MD (Multidisciplinary Association for Psychedelic Studies 2019)

PEAT: Primordial Energy Activation and Transcendence and the Neutralization of Polarities by Zivorad Slavinski (Arelena Publishing, 2007) *Return to Oneness: Principles and Practice of Spiritual Technology* by Zivorad Slavinski (AuthorHouse, 2009)

Bondassage: Kinky Erotic Massage Tips for Lovers by Jaeleen Bennis and Eve Minax (Dymaxicon, 2013)

The Deepest Acceptance: Radical Awakening in Ordinary Life by Jeff Foster (Sounds True, 2012)

Women's Anatomy of Arousal: Secret Maps to Buried Pleasure by Sheri Winston (Mango Garden Press, 2011)

Other Online Resources

The Sexual Excitation/Sexual Inhibition Inventory for Women: Psychometric Properties, kinseyinstitute.org/pdf/Factoranalysis.pdf

This is a paper about the inventory. The surveys are meant to be administered by clinical professionals. A self-administered version can be found in Emily Nagoski's book *Come As You Are,* pp. 54–57.

Sex Education for Emerging Adults

SCARLETEEN
scarleteen.com

I often get asked by parents how they can help their teens learn more about healthy sexuality. This website provides inclusive, comprehensive, and supportive sex education and relationship information for teens and emerging adults.

Music Playlists Themed for the Blueprint Types

On Spotify: Search for *TheEcstaticLife*
Find many playlists broken down by Blueprint Types.

Helping Professionals

Sex-Positive Therapists

ESTHER PEREL
estherperel.com

Esther Perel has been an inspiration, mentor, guide, and friend for over a decade. She is one of the most brilliant women I know. As a therapist and world-renowned speaker, she helps people around the globe build a healthy eroticism.

CARISTA LUMINARE, PHD

confusedaboutlove.com

Carista Luminare is a skillful guide and counselor with over forty years of experience helping couples create healthy attachment bonds. She wisely works on many layers and dynamics in relationships.

KATE LOREE

www.kateloree.squarespace.com

Kate Loree was our go-to sex-positive and kink-friendly therapist, and helped Ian and me navigate challenging terrain when we started to expand into the Kinky Blueprint. With a hugely compassionate heart and creative style, she helps people find healing.

Mentors, Coaches, Guides, and Practitioners

JAIYA—PRIVATE MENTORSHIP

JaiyaMentorships.com

I offer private, yearlong bespoke mentorships with immersive luxury retreats to erotic seekers who desire access to empowered sexual freedom and an awakening to their True Self.

IAN FERGUSON—COACH

ecstasislab.com

Besides being my sexy lover, Ian is my cocreator of the Erotic Blueprint Breakthrough and CEO of the Blueprint Breakthrough, Inc. As a coach, he helps clients manifest their ideal vision for their lives, especially in the areas of relationship, expression, and abundance. His live workshops also use interactive games, music, movement, and practices to help people experience flow state and greater personal freedom.

CHRISTIAN DUHAMEL—INTIMACY, EXPRESSION, AND VOICE COACH

cobalt-phoenix.com

One of my favorite humans on this planet! Christian is an internationally regarded playwright, lyricist, composer, actor, voice teacher, and voice coach, and is the founder of Cobalt Phoenix. As an artist, teacher, and mentor, he is passionate about helping people discover and develop their authentic voices as they explore the dynamic intersection of intimacy, creativity, and self-growth.

JOSEPH KRAMER, PHD—MENTOR

eroticmassage.com

Joseph Kramer truly transformed the trajectory of my career and deeply contributed to the creation of the field of somatic sexology. As the creator Sexological Bodywork, he is a trailblazer for embodied sexuality education.

KENNETH RAY STUBBS—MENTOR

therainbowbody.com

I feel so much affection when I think of this being. Kenneth Ray Stubbs has been a guide and mentor to me, and a shining light for the world. If you are interested in Energetic expansion, be sure to visit his body of work.

SATYEN AND SUZANNE RAJA—MENTORS AND COACHES

warriorsage.com

Satyen and Suzanne Raja have been mentors to Ian and me, guiding us in many facets of life, love, business, and spirituality. They are leaders to other leaders, helping them grow into authentic truth. Satyen is also the founder of Accelerated Evolution Academy.

WESLY FEUQUAY—MENTOR AND TEACHER

weslyfeuquay.com

Wesly Feuquay is a mentor and teacher who works with psychospiritual processes to help people heal, transform, and awaken. He helps people live from the truth of deeper knowing that we all possess.

ELLEN HEED, PHD—SCAR TISSUE REMEDIATION, EDUCATION, AND MANAGEMENT

scartissueremediation.com

Ellen Heed's work and mentorship in scar tissue remediation truly saved my sexuality after the birth of my son. She has created an entire body of work and trains other practitioners to help people heal from scar-related physical, emotional, and unseen trauma.

ORI ZIMMELS—MENTOR, PHILOSOPHER, AND GUIDE

lifeawake.com

Ori specializes in the exploration and access of internal and somatic states. Through curiosity and permission, he helps people discover purpose and meaning, and develop a deeper and more consistent sense of self. He is also dedicated to helping those who seek to awaken in this lifetime.

BODHI AVINASHA—FOUNDER OF IPSALU TANTRA

ipsalutantra.org

Bodhi Avinasha, a founder of Ipsalu Tantra, was one of my first mentors in Tantric sexuality. If you are curious about the Transformational stage of sexuality or

Energetic expansion, Ipsalu is a great place to start.

ORPHEUS BLACK—KINK EDUCATOR AND PRACTITIONER
orpheusblack.com

The boundless ocean of spiritual and sensual exploration finds expression through Orpheus Black's offerings, blending the depths of kink with the heights of sacred masculinity and femininity. With wisdom as vast as the heavens and earth, he guides seekers through themes of psychosensuality and archetypal psychology, leading them, in his classes, workshops, retreats, and private coaching, to a deeper understanding of themselves and the profound intimacy of healthy expressions of Dominance and submission.

JAELEEN BENNIS—KINK EDUCATOR AND FOUNDER OF BONDASSAGE
jaeleenbennis.com

Jaeleen Bennis is a wise, beautiful soul and the creator of Bondassage, which to me is the poetic dance between the Kinky and Sensual Blueprints. She is a mentor to many and another pioneer who deeply inspires erotic players to play full out!

Doctors for Hormone Health

DR. PRUDENCE HALL
The Hall Center
thehallcenter.com

I had the great opportunity to work with Dr. Prudence Hall after the birth of my son. She is a caring, brilliant woman who understands the Biochemical realm and helps others optimize their sexual health and longevity.

DR. DAVID TUSEK
cloudmedical.io

Dr. Tusek and Cloud Medical are another resource for all things related to your sexual health in all realms. They look at the person as a whole being and take a well-rounded approach that includes your biochemistry.

Podcasts

LIFE AWAKE: CONTEMPLATIVE SHORTS WITH JAIYA AND ORI ZIMMELS
lifeawake.com/podcasts.html

Welcome to my new podcast, where Ori and I explore "Contemplative Shorts," which are expressions of wisdom condensed into short form. All are aimed at being passages toward awakening, leading us closer to our authentic self and the discovery of our deeper truth. With this comes the blossoming of consciousness and the revelation of unity.

Helpful Organizations

MAPS (MULTIDISCIPLINARY ASSOCIATION FOR PSYCHEDELIC STUDIES)
maps.org/our-research

As a nonprofit research center working in the field of psychedelics, MAPS has truly transformed the lives of those suffering with mental health challenges such as PTSD, anxiety disorders, and depression. They are at the forefront of the legalization of these breakthrough therapies.

REGENESIS SANCTUARY—ADDICTION RECOVERY
regenesissanctuary.com

My cofounders and I created Regenesis Sanctuary to offer a private, bespoke solution to the growing problem of addiction. Using an exclusive, world-class protocol, our dedicated team guides you on the path to the most fulfilled version of yourself.

ACCELERATED EVOLUTION ACADEMY: ELIMINATING EMOTIONAL BLOCKS
acceleratedevolutionacademy.com

Accelerated Evolution Academy is an organization aimed at helping people create lasting transformation through processes that quickly remove emotional distress. Most Erotic Blueprint coaches and I are trained in these methodologies.

HOLOTROPIC BREATHWORK
holotropic.com

Created by Stanislav Grof, Holotropic Breathwork was designed to help people return to wholeness. I recommend finding a practitioner near you if you are interested in accessing expanded states of consciousness, transpersonal psychology, and the Energetic Blueprint.

Legal

NATIONAL COALITION FOR SEXUAL FREEDOM (NCSF)
ncsfreedom.org

NCSF is a nonprofit that advocates for people who identify as Kinky and nonmonogamous. Since 1997 they have worked to destigmatize and provide education about BDSM and polyamory.

DIANA ADAMS LAW & MEDIATION, PLLC

DianaAdamsLaw.net

Diana does mediation for polyamorous families and works on non-legal agreements internationally and throughout the US, and provides state-specific legal advice only in New York. They are part of leadership in an international network of LGBTQ+ lawyers and can offer referral for international colleagues.

Emergency Hotlines

If you are in immediate danger, call 9-1-1.

For less urgent matters:

NATIONAL COALITION AGAINST DOMESTIC VIOLENCE

ncadv.org/get-help

For anonymous, confidential help, 24-7, please call the National Domestic Violence Hotline at 1-800-799-7233.

THE TREVOR PROJECT

thetrevorproject.org

The Trevor Project provides information and support to LGBTQ+ young people, 24-7.

notes

CHAPTER THREE
Who Are We? Erotic Blueprints Are Born

31   Jack Morin's concepts "Core Erotic Themes" and "Peak Erotic Experiences" inspired Jaiya's creation of the Erotic Blueprints. J. Morin, *The Erotic Mind* (HarperCollins, 1995).

CHAPTER FOUR
Erotic Myths

42   *Inadequate sex education, combined with over a century of sexuality research focused primarily on dysfunction, has created a lot of unnecessary suffering around our sex lives*: We refer to the field of sex research as sexology. It is the scientific study of sexual behavior. In the late nineteenth century, scholars in Germany, Austria, and Britain pioneered this research. French philosopher Michel Foucault, the author of *The History of Sexuality: An Introduction* (1978), criticized the science of sex by saying that sex is managed by doctors influenced by politics to enforce social norms and not so much to cure health problems. He believed that early sexual science did not provide the truth of sex by promoting health, but instead, sexology was used to normalize the monogamous, heterosexual nuclear family.

45   *Problems with low sexual desire or SDD are one of the most common causes of distress in relationships, and are the primary reason couples go to see a sex therapist*: P. J. Kleinplatz et al., "From Sexual Desire Discrepancies to Desirable Sex: Creating the Optimal Connection," *Journal of Sex and Marital Therapy* 44, no. 5 (2018): 438–449, https://doi.org/10.1080/0092623x.2017.1405309.

45   *Canadian clinical psychologist and sexologist Peggy J. Kleinplatz
has spent decades investigating what makes up "optimal sexual
experiences."*: Peggy J. Kleinplatz and A. Ménard, *Magnificent Sex:
Lessons from Extraordinary Lovers* (Routledge, 2020).

48   *In their 1973 book* Sexual Conduct, *sociologists John Gagnon and
William Simon first introduced sexual scripts theory as a framework
for understanding sexual interactions and scenarios*: J. Gagnon and
W. Simon, *Sexual Conduct: The Social Origins of Human Sexuality*
(Chicago: Aldine, 1973).

52   *SCT challenged the ideas that gender is binary and sexual attraction
is only based on gender."*: S. M. van Anders, "Beyond Sexual
Orientation: Integrating Gender/Sex and Diverse Sexualities via Sexual
Configurations Theory," *Archives of Sexual Behavior* 44, no. 5 (2015):
1177–1213, https://doi.org/10.1007/s10508-015-0490-8; A. Iantaffi and
M.-J. Barker, "Mapping Your Sexuality: From Sexual Orientation to
Sexual Configurations Theory," https://www.rewriting-the-rules.com/
sex/new-zine-mapping-your-sexuality.

CHAPTER FIVE
Five Stages of Sexuality: Which One Are You Living In?

66   *The World Health Organization (WHO) estimated that worldwide,
approximately 13 percent of people aged fifteen to forty-nine had HSV-2
(herpes simplex virus type 2) in 2022*: World Health Organization,
"Herpes Simplex Virus," March 10, 2022, https://www.who.int/
news-room/fact-sheets/detail/herpes-simplex-virus.

67   *The Centers for Disease Control and Prevention estimated that 12 percent of
people aged fourteen to forty-nine had HSV-2 infection in the United States
as of 2018*: Centers for Disease Control and Prevention, "Detailed Std Facts
- Genital Herpes," June 28, 2022, https://www.cdc.gov/std/herpes/stdfact-
herpes-detailed.htm#ref1.

CHAPTER SEVEN
The Energetic

102   *The work of Stanislav Grof, a brilliant psychiatrist and pioneer in
transpersonal psychiatry, may explain a lot of what Energetics
experience*: S. Grof, "Dr. Stanislav Grof," https://www.stangrof.com.

102   *"My consciousness expanded at an inconceivable speed and reached
cosmic dimensions. I lost connection with my everyday identity . . . I
became everything.":* S. Grof, *The Way of the Psychonaut: Encyclopedia
for Inner Journeys*, vol. 1, 1st ed. (Multidisciplinary Association for
Psychedelic Studies, 2019); Grof and S. Grof, "Spiritual Emergency: The
Understanding and Treatment of Transpersonal Crises," *International
Journal of Transpersonal Studies* 36, no. 2 (2017): 30–43, https://doi.
org/10.24972/ijts.2017.36.2.30.

103   *Biomagnetics is the study of magnetic fields produced by living
organisms:* J. L. Oschman, *Energy Medicine: The Scientific Basis*, 2nd ed.
(Elsevier, 2016).

CHAPTER EIGHT
The Sensual

117   *Hypervigilance is an elevated state where we perceive that there may
be some kind of danger or potential threat around us, even when there
isn't:* A. K. Randall and G. Bodenmann, "The Role of Stress on Close
Relationships and Marital Satisfaction," *Clinical Psychology Review* 29,
no. 2 (2009): 105–115, https://doi.org/10.1016/j.cpr.2008.10.004.

119   *Some of these include exposure to cold, slow diaphragmatic breathing,
meditation, vocalization (singing, humming, gargling, and laughing),
and, exciting for us, sexual intercourse:* "Vagus Nerve Stimulation,"
Wim Hof Method, 2023, https://www.wimhofmethod.com/vagus-nerve-
stimulation; R. J. Ellis and J. F. Thayer, "Music and Autonomic Nervous
System (Dys)Function," *Music Perception* 27, no. 4 (2010): 317.

121   *He told me about a study from Lucia Benetti which demonstrated that
some babies even sing before they speak, repeating simple melodies,
the lyrics to which they can't yet understand or pronounce the lyrics:* L.
Benetti and E. Costa-Giomi, "Infant Vocal Imitation of Music," *Journal
of Research in Music Education* 67, no. 4 (2020): 381–398, https://doi.
org/10.1177/0022429419890328.

CHAPTER NINE
The Sexual

136   *Some Sexuals may wonder if they have a "sex addiction.":* B. Reay,
N. Attwood, and C. Gooder, "Inventing Sex: The Short History of

Sex Addiction," *Sexuality & Culture* 17, no. 1 (2012): 1–19, https://doi. org/10.1007/s12119-012-9136-3.

137   *In relationships, the "sex addict" label tends to be placed on the person who wants more intercourse than their partner*: American Association of Sexuality Educators, Counselors and Therapists, "AASECT Position on Sex Addiction," last modified 2016, https://www.aasect.org/ position-sex-addiction.

137   *According to the World Health Organization, compulsive sexual behavior disorder is diagnosed when a person's sexual impulses and urges are so intense, they are unable to control their behavior*: World Health Organization, "6C72 Compulsive Sexual Behaviour Disorder," ICD-11 for Mortality and Morbidity Statistics (January 2023), accessed March 2, 2023, https://icd.who.int/browse11/l-m/en#/http%253A%252F%252Fid. who.int%252Ficd%252Fentity%252F1630268048.

140   *She says that guilt is when we say to ourselves "I've done something wrong or bad." And shame is when we say to ourselves "I am bad.":* B. Brown, *The Gifts of Imperfection: Let Go of Who You Think You're Supposed to Be and Embrace Who You Are*, 1st ed. (Hazelden Publishing, 2010).

140   *Babies in the womb stimulate their own genitals*: I. Meizner, "Sonographic Observation of In Utero Fetal 'Masturbation,'" *Journal of Ultrasound in Medicine* 6, no. 2 (1987): 111, https://doi.org/10.7863/ jum.1987.6.2.111.

CHAPTER TEN
The Kinky

154   *My friend Jaeleen Bennis, creator of Bondassage, says that you can make anything a "pervertible!":* https://bondassage.com.

156   *Research shows that kinky people do not suffer from mental illness to a greater extent than the general population*: C. R. Dunkley and L. A. Brotto, "Clinical Considerations in Treating BDSM Practitioners: A Review," *Journal of Sex & Marital Therapy* 44, no. 7 (2018): 701–712, https://doi.org/10.1080/0092623x.2018.1451792.

156   *But several major research studies have concluded that people who engage in and enjoy kink aren't more likely to have a history of trauma*

or mental illness: J. Richters et al., "Demographic and Psychosocial Features of Participants in Bondage and Discipline, 'Sadomasochism' or Dominance and Submission (BDSM): Data from a National Survey," *Journal of Sexual Medicine* 5, no. 7 (2008): 1660–1668, https://doi.org/10.1111/j.1743-6109.2008.00795.x; A. A. Wismeijer and M. A. van Assen, "Psychological Characteristics of BDSM Practitioners," *Journal of Sexual Medicine* 10, no. 8 (2013): 1943–1952, https://doi.org/10.1111/jsm.12192.

156   *Kink is also empowering to people who have a history of trauma, and can help navigate past experiences of powerlessness, embarrassment, discomfort, and stress*: B. L. Simula, "Pleasure, Power, and Pain: A Review of the Literature on the Experiences of BDSM Participants," *Sociology Compass* 13, no. 3 (2019): 1–24, https://doi.org/10.1111/soc4.12668.

156   *A 2018 study from Richard Sprott and Bren Hadcock of bisexual, pansexual, and queer kink participants found that kink activities can have many uses . . .*: R. A. Sprott and B. B. Hadcock, "Bisexuality, Pansexuality, Queer Identity, and Kink Identity," *Sexual and Relationship Therapy* 33, no. 1–2 (2018): 214–232, https://doi.org/10.1080/14681994.2017.1347616.

157   *As a matter of fact, studies have shown that people who are Kinky, and have cultivated conscientious expressions of their kinky desires . . .*: A. A. Wismeijer and M. A. van Assen, "Psychological Characteristics of BDSM Practitioners," *Journal of Sexual Medicine* 10, no. 8 (2013): 1943–1952, https://doi.org/10.1111/jsm.12192; A. Hébert and A. Weaver, "An Examination of Personality Characteristics Associated with BDSM Orientations," *Canadian Journal of Human Sexuality* 23, no. 2 (2014): 106–115, https://doi.org/10.3138/cjhs.2467.

159   *The American Psychiatric Association removed consensual BDSM . . . and fetish play from the DSM in 2013*: American Psychiatric Association, "Paraphilic Disorders," in *Diagnostic and Statistical Manual of Mental Disorders*, 5th ed. (American Psychiatric Publishing, 2013).

164   *According to research, pain feels good during kinky experiences because it involves the pleasure and reward systems . . .*: E. Wuyts and M. Morrens, "The Biology of BDSM: A Systematic Review," *Journal of Sexual Medicine* 19, no. 1 (2022): 144–157, https://doi.org/10.1016/j.jsxm.2021.11.002.

166   *In 2019, a group of sexuality researchers theorized why pain might be experienced as pleasurable among those who practice BDSM*: C. R. Dunkley et al., "Physical Pain as Pleasure: A Theoretical Perspective," *Journal of Sex Research* 57, no. 4 (2019): 421–437, https://doi.org/10.1080/00224499.2019.1605328.

CHAPTER TWELVE
Determining Erotic Blueprints

193   *Evolving research indicates that practicing mindfulness-based exercises like this may be very effective in restoring connectivity to the brain's networks*: J. E. Boyd, R. A. Lanius, and M. C. McKinnon, "Mindfulness-Based Treatments for Posttraumatic Stress Disorder: A Review of the Treatment Literature and Neurobiological Evidence," *Journal of Psychiatry & Neuroscience* 43, no. 1 (2018): 7–25, https://doi.org/10.1503/jpn.170021.

207   *Research indicates that people with higher levels of the stress hormone cortisol tend to experience lower levels of sexual desire, sexual activity, sexual satisfaction, and sexual pleasure*: American Psychological Association, "Stress Effects on the Body," APA, November 1, 2018, https://www.apa.org/topics/stress/body; G. Bodenmann et al., "The Association between Daily Stress and Sexual Activity," *Journal of Family Psychology* 24, no. 3 (2010): 271–279, https://doi.org/10.1037/a0019365.

CHAPTER FOURTEEN
The Four Obstacles to Sexual Health and Pleasure

235   *According to research, most doctors don't ask their patients about sexual problems, sexual satisfaction, or pleasure*: J. N. Sobecki et al., "What We Don't Talk about When We Don't Talk about Sex: Results of a National Survey of U.S. Obstetrician/Gynecologists," *Journal of Sexual Medicine* 9, no. 5 (2012): 1285–1294, https://doi.org/10.1111/j.1743-6109.2012.02702.x.

235   *A 2018 survey found only half of the medical schools in the United States required formal instruction in sexuality*: C. Warner et al., "Sexual Health Knowledge of U.S. Medical Students: A National Survey," *Journal of Sexual Medicine* 15, no. 8 (2018): 1093–1102, https://doi.org/10.1016/j.jsxm.2018.05.019.

238 *Almost three out of every four women experience pain during intercourse at some point in their lifetime*: American College of Obstetricians and Gynecologists, "When Sex Is Painful," ACOG, January 2022, https://www.acog.org/womens-health/faqs/when-sex-is-painful?utm_source=redirect%26utm_medium=web&utm_campaign=otn#how.

238 *An estimated 30 to 50 million men in the United States and 150 million men worldwide experience ED*: T. Sooriyamoorthy and S. W. Leslie, "Erectile Dysfunction," StatPearls (May 27, 2022), retrieved October 3, 2022, from https://www.ncbi.nlm.nih.gov/books/NBK562253.

238 *A meta-analysis of fourteen studies involving over ninety thousand men with ED revealed that they had 44 percent more cardiovascular events, 62 percent more heart attacks, 39 percent more strokes, and a 25 percent higher risk of death compared to patients who did not have ED*: C. V. Vlachopoulos et al., "Prediction of Cardiovascular Events and All-Cause Mortality with Erectile Dysfunction," *Circulation: Cardiovascular Quality and Outcomes* 6, no. 1 (2013): 99–109, https://doi.org/10.1161/circoutcomes.112.966903.

240 *I have found that the best processes for clearing emotional charges are those created by Zivorad Slavinski . . .*: Z. Slavinski, *PEAT: Primordial Energy Activation and Transcendence and the Neutralization of Polarities* (Arelena Publishing, 2007); Slavinski, *Return to Oneness: Principles and Practice of Spiritual Technology* (AuthorHouse, 2009).·

243 *The bioelectrical flows produced by organs such as the heart, brain, and muscles are the most well-documented energy fields . . .*: J. L. Oschman, *Energy Medicine: The Scientific Basis*, 2nd ed. (Elsevier, 2016).

246 *The "accelerator and brakes" model was first popularized by Emily Nagoski in her book* Come As You Are: E. Nagoski, *Come As You Are: The Surprising New Science That Will Transform Your Sex Life*, revised ed. (Simon & Schuster, 2021).

246 *The Dual Control Model, developed in the late 1990s at the Kinsey Institute, is the current theoretical model of sexual response today*: Kinsey Institute, "Dual Control Model of Sexual Response," n.d., https://kinseyinstitute.org/research/dual-control-model.php.

256   *Her ACE (Adverse Childhood Experience) score was an 8 out of 10, which is very high*: Centers for Disease Control and Prevention, "Adverse Childhood Experiences (ACEs)," https://www.cdc.gov/violenceprevention/aces/index.html.

CHAPTER SIXTEEN
Feeding, Speaking, Healing, and Expanding Your Erotic Blueprint

272   *Boost immune function: Sex significantly raises your levels of immunoglobulin A (IgA), an important antibody that is part of your immune system*: C. J. Charnetski and F. X. Brennan, "Sexual Frequency and Salivary Immunoglobulin A (IgA)," *Psychological Reports* 94, no. 3 (2004): 839–844, https://doi.org/10.2466/pr0.94.3.839-844.

272   *Better aging: One study found that feelings of well-being are higher among older adults who are sexually active*: L. Smith et al., "Sexual Activity Is Associated with Greater Enjoyment of Life in Older Adults," *Sexual Medicine* 7, no. 1 (2019): 11–18, https://doi.org/10.1016/j.esxm.2018.11.001.

272   *Better sleep: Orgasm increases levels of prolactin and oxytocin, hormones that promote sleep and relaxation, so having sex may make it easier to fall asleep*: M. Lastella et al., "Sex and Sleep: Perceptions of Sex as a Sleep Promoting Behavior in the General Adult Population," *Frontiers in Public Health* 7 (2019), https://doi.org/10.3389/fpubh.2019.00033.

exercise index

about the author

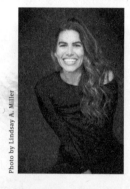

Photo by Lindsay A. Miller

JAIYA has spent close to three decades on a mission to help erotic seekers transform sexual shame into freedom and suffering into awakening. She is the cofounder of the Erotic Blueprint Breakthrough, the author of multiple bestselling books, and a mentor to award-winning celebrities, Olympic athletes, high-net-worth leaders, and entrepreneurs.

Jaiya helps high performers create a pleasure-filled life so that instead of running themselves and their relationships into the grave, they can live life from a place of embodied peak existence. She is dedicated to a world where love is awakened in all our hearts. Jaiya has recently started several philanthropic endeavors to help all of humanity have their basic human needs met and to help awaken higher consciousness on this planet.